How to Start an Independent Practice

The Nurse Practitioner's Guide to Success

Carolyn Zaumeyer MSN, ARNP

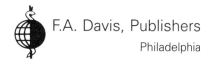

F.A. Davis, Publishers

Philadelphia

F. A. Davis Company
1915 Arch Street
Philadelphia, PA 19103
www.fadavis.com

Printed in the United States of America

Last digit indicates print number: 10 9 8 7 6 5 4 3 2 1

Acquisitions Editor: Joanne Patzek DaCunha, RN, MSN
Developmental Editor: Marilyn Kochman
Cover Designer: Louis J. Forgione

As new scientific information becomes available through basic and clinical research, recommended treatments and drug therapies undergo changes. The author(s) and publisher have done everything possible to make this book accurate, up to date, and in accord with accepted standards at the time of publication. The author(s), editors, and publisher are not responsible for errors or omissions or for consequences from application of the book, and make no warranty, expressed or implied, in regard to the contents of the book. Any practice described in this book should be applied by the reader in accordance with professional standards of care used in regard to the unique circumstances that may apply in each situation. The reader is advised always to check product information (package inserts) for changes and new information regarding dose and contraindications before administering any drug. Caution is especially urged when using new or infrequently ordered drugs.

Library of Congress Cataloging-in-Publication Data

Zaumeyer, Carolyn R.
  How to start an independent practice : the nurse practitioner's guide to success /
Carolyn R. Zaumeyer.
      p. ; cm.
  Includes bibliographical references and index.
  ISBN 0-8036-1058-0
    1. Nurse practitioners—Practice. 2. New business enterprises—Management. I. Title.
  [DNLM: 1. Nurse Practitioners—organization & administration. 2.
  Entrepreneurship—organization & administration. 3. Private Practice—organization &
  administration. WY 128 Z39h 2003]
  RT86.7.Z38 2003
  610.73′06′92—dc21

                                                                          2003043772

To my favorite husband Chuck, whose kindness and humor make me smile every day.

To my parents, for their never-ending support and their belief in my ability to succeed (and also for their editing skills!).

To David, Gwen, Jock, Mary Ellen, and Kristen for their interest, insight and suggestions.

To Butkus and Cuff for their companionship, conversation and paws on my keyboard when I had been working for too many hours.

Preface

In January 1994 I established an independent practice in Ft. Lauderdale, Florida, *Women's Health Watch, Inc.* Before starting the practice I did extensive research and was unable to locate a good resource written specifically for nurse practitioners interested in independent practice. After I established my practice and could see that I was on the road to success, I decided that I could share my new knowledge and help other nurse practitioners to realize their dream too. I wrote my first book *The Nurse Practitioner as Entrepreneur: How to Establish and Operate an Independent Practice*, in 1995. The book has enjoyed great success as a textbook as well as a resource and reference manual for nurse practitioners. Now it is time for a more comprehensive and current manual for nurse practitioners interested in independent practice.

Many nurse practitioners harbor the dream of establishing and operating an independent practice. Many people have tried to identify the specific personality traits of the successful entrepreneur. Do you have the "E" or entrepreneurial personality? Some questions you may ask of yourself include: Am I a leader? Am I self-motivated? Do I have good people skills? Am I goal-oriented? Do I have the skills necessary? Do I have a creative mind? Do I have an optimistic outlook on life? Am I mentally, physically, and financially ready for this venture?

This book takes you from helping you make the decision whether to open your own practice through the specifics of how to put your practice together. Once you have put your practice together, you will need to know how to run it on a day-to-day basis. Marketing is a major factor in growing a successful business. Included you will find many interesting marketing concepts and unique ideas to promote your practice. The final chapter gives information on how to sell your practice so you will be prepared if you get a great offer!

All of this may sound overwhelming, but by following the guidelines provided you can break down the tasks necessary for success into workable sections. Breaking the process of starting your own practice down into step-by-step actions can help you make your dreams come true.

Many nurse practitioner programs do not include business courses in their curriculum. Whether you chose to open your own practice or not, having a good understanding of the business of the practice is imperative to practice professionally as a nurse practitioner. As an entrepreneur there are many business strategies to grasp. My intention with this text is to provide the entrepreneurial nurse practitioner with information to guide you through the process of establishing and operating an independent practice.

Good luck!

CAROLYN ZAUMEYER

Consultants

Janet Geare Allen, RN, MSN, PHN, CHPN
Full Time Administrator of Hospice and Palliative Care Program
Kaiser Permanente
Downey, California

Jean Krajicek Bartek, Ph.D, APRN
Associate Professor
University of Nebraska Medical Center
Colleges of Nursing, and Medicine (Pharmacology)
Omaha, Nebraska

Barbara Mathews Blanton, MSN, RN, CARN
Assistant Clinical Professor
Texas Woman's University
Dallas, Texas

Barbara Brush, RNC, PhD, FAAN
Associate Professor
William F. Connell School of Nursing
Boston College
Chestnut Hill, Massachusetts

Dolores W. Clark, RN, FNP, CPNP
Acting Director, Pediatric Nurse Practitioner Program
University of Texas
Arlington, Texas

M. Katherine Crabtree, RN, DNSc, APRN, BC
Professor
Oregon Health and Sciences University
Portland, Oregon

Amy Sedlacek Cooper, BSN, MSN
Research Nurse Practitioner
Womens and Infants' Hospital, Division of Research
Providence, Rhode Island

Brenda Drummond, MSN, CNP, CNS
Owner, Practitioner
Nurse Practitioner Consultants, LLC
Perrysburg, Ohio
Doctoral Student
University of Michigan School of Nursing
Ann Arbor, Michigan

Holly Kennedy, PhD, CNM, FACNM
Assistant Professor and Director
University of Rhode Island
Kingston, Rhode Island

Nanette Lavoie-Vaughan, MSN, ARNP-C
Former CEO
Housecall Physicians
Raleigh, North Carolina

Susanne J. Phillips, MSN, ARNP, BC, FNP
Part-Time Faculty
University of California, Irvine
School of Medicine
Department of Family Medicine
Family Nurse Practitioner Education
Irvine, California

Marilyn Smith-Stoner, RN, PhD
Faculty
California State University
Fullerton, California
Co-Owner
Power Components
Mentone, California

Pat Woodbery, BSN, MSN, ARNP-CS
Professor of Nursing
Valencia Community College
Orlando, Florida

Contents

Before You Start Your Practice

Chapter 1

Personal Considerations: Should I Start an Independent Practice?

" Our aspirations are our possibilities "

Robert Browning

D eciding to start your own practice may be one of the most significant decisions you make in your lifetime. It could bring you great fulfillment and happiness, or, in some cases, great worry and hardship. This is *not* a decision to take lightly.

ASSESSING THE DEMANDS

One of the first steps in determining whether or not independent practice is for you is to perform a self-assessment. There is no better place to start than by assessing your own goals, strengths, and weaknesses:

- Evaluate your own personal desires. Do *you* really want to do this, or are others pressuring you to start your own practice?
- Look at your financial situation: Can you afford to possibly live without a paycheck for a couple of years?
- Consider your family situation. Will your family support you? The heavy demands of owning and operating a practice will surely impact your family life.

Think about this thoroughly. What do *you* want to do with your life and your career?

The extent of your business knowledge must be addressed. If you do not have a strong business background, find people to help you. Recognizing your strengths and weaknesses in business knowledge helps you identify areas where you may want to consult other professionals—attorneys, accountants, marketing specialists.

Remember the "care plans" we used to prepare for our patients in nursing school? Preparing for entrepreneurship can be handled in the same manner. Set both personal and business goals for both the short term and the long term. Where do you want to be 1 year from now? In 5 years? Even in the next 10 years? Write down the answers—it is interesting to look back over the years at your goals. No matter what your motivation is to start a practice, setting both personal and business goals not only helps in the decision making but also lays the foundation for your future business. One of the best ways to determine your personal and business goals is to list them on the following worksheet (Fig. 1–1). List both your personal and professional goals for 1, 5, and 10 years. Make your goals realistic, attainable, and measurable.

No matter what type of practice you wish to open, you must take a serious look at your life situation before you make your decision. Business ownership is not for everyone and not all business ideas are viable. You may have a concept that sounds great to you and your friends, but you must complete the research and planning process to know whether you will be able to develop a profitable practice.

Many people who have the motivation and desire for business ownership have failed because they have not taken the time to properly evaluate their business concept. Consider your practice style—Do you like to work on your own or are you more comfortable with another professional in the same office? Do you think you could continue to grow as a practitioner on your own? Would you feel better with a partner? Some people are just not cut out for independent practice—and that's okay! There are plenty of work situations for those most comfortable practicing with other professionals.

Is independent practice for you? That is the real question. Examine why you want to start a practice and whether you have the personal qualities needed for a demanding professional situation:

- Do you feel comfortable with the sacrifices you will have to make as a business owner?
- Do you have the support of your family, friends, and colleagues?
- Do you have the desire to confront the many risks associated with opening a business?
- Do you enjoy working autonomously?

Only after a thorough evaluation of topics such as these should you continue on with the planning process for starting your own practice.

Figure 1-1 Setting Personal and Business Goals.

	1 YEAR	5 YEARS	10 YEARS

PERSONAL GOAL #1

PERSONAL GOAL #2

PERSONAL GOAL #3

BUSINESS GOAL #1

BUSINESS GOAL #2

BUSINESS GOAL #3

CHARACTERISTICS OF BUSINESS SUCCESS AND FAILURE

It has been estimated that more than fifty percent of new businesses fail within the first few years of business. There are numerous risks associated with becoming an entrepreneur. One of the main reasons given for the high failure rate is that many businesses have been built primarily on desire and have neglected the critical building blocks of competence and planning. Don't let this happen to you.

Numerous texts on the subject indicate that lack of financing or undercapitalization is the primary reason for failure. However, a literature review on small business ownership indicates that the majority of new business failures are due to either a lack of business competence or a lack of management experience, or both. According to the literature, this lack of competence is usually due to one or more of the following:

- Poor planning
- Inadequate market analysis
- Product problems and defects
- Lack of proper marketing and advertising
- Poor start-up timing
- Failure to anticipate the competition
- Unanticipated costs
- Continuous shortage of funds
- Failure to keep proper financial records
- Failure to keep up with industry trends
- Inadequate inventory control
- Poor control of credit

Make a note card with the points on this list that could affect your business and put it in a place where you will see it on a regular basis. You must stay on top of these things. You do not want to become a failure statistic.

Starting a business is similar to playing with building blocks. You have to build one block at a time. If you plan each action as you build each segment of your new venture, you will build a strong foundation for your business. This process dramatically enhances your chances of success.

Evaluating your personal and business goals that you have listed will help you visualize your practice and will aid you in the process of developing your practice. Remember that you do not have to build your practice on your own.

There are many professionals who can help you in areas in which you are not familiar. You do not have to be an expert in business to start a practice, but you must have a realistic understanding of your own strengths and weaknesses. If you identify an area where you need help, you can compensate for that weakness and turn it into a strength.

Over time, expertise can be learned or bought. In other words, if you have a particular weakness, you can compensate for that weakness by taking classes, hiring staff, or retaining consultants. Numerous workshops offer assistance on various topics regarding business ownership. You do not need to know everything about everything, but you must have a good overview of the running of your practice. Ultimately, you are responsible for all aspects of your business. Using the following Strengths and Weaknesses worksheet (Fig. 1–2), list your own personal strengths and weaknesses as they relate to your desire to open an independent practice. In identifying strengths and weaknesses, consider education, experience, personal quirks, and overall business knowledge. Specifically include your strengths and weaknesses in the following areas:

- Overall business knowledge
- Marketing and promotion
- Business finance
- Business management
- Organizational skills
- Work habits
- Motivation
- Leadership skills
- Personal fears or obstacles
- Target markets
- Business monitoring
- Record keeping
- Insurance regulations and needs
- Legal documents and requirements
- Publicity and public relations
- Ability to establish short-term and long-term objectives
- Personal situation including family, finances, and business demands

Much has been written about the personal qualities of the successful entrepreneur. Particularly, they are highly motivated, possess strong leadership skills, are hard working, and plan before they act. After you identify your personal strengths and weaknesses on Figure 1–2, draft an initial action plan, which will help you as you develop your new business.

Figure 1-2 Strengths and Weaknesses

Strengths	Weaknesses	Action Plan	Time and Charges

A summary of your personal strengths and weaknesses will help highlight your "state of readiness" as it pertains to your goal of establishing a practice as an entrepreneur.

Strengths   =   List any personal strengths you have at the present time.

Weaknesses   =   Specify any weaknesses that may hinder your progress.

Action Plan   =   Possible methods of dealing with your specified weaknesses.

Time and Charges =   Concerning your Action Plan, list any cost involved and the time required for implementation.

THE SIGNIFICANCE OF RESEARCH AND PLANNING

Now that you have assessed your own personal strengths and weaknesses, as well as the demands of independent practice, it is crucial that you seriously research or investigate your ideas as a means of developing your concept into a reality. Many people skip this important step and those are usually the people who fail. You must take the time to truly define and develop your practice.

The next step is to continue on building the foundation of your practice by outlining the type, size and scope of your proposed practice. For example, you may consider:

What type of practice do you intend to establish?

What services will be provided?

Where will your practice be located?

How many employees will you need?

What distinguishes your proposed practice from others?

Is there really a need for your practice in the community?

In short, your purpose in this stage of development is to describe your proposed new practice, being as specific as possible.

Your business decisions should be based on fact, not fancy. Therefore, as you mold your practice, start by listing all the information you will need to help you make informed decisions. The Internet has endless information available on all subjects of business. Other sources include: textbooks, seminars, teachers, consultants, government organizations, trade publications and organizations—even friends and family. And don't forget the Yellow Pages. One of the first steps I took when researching the feasibility of opening Women's Health Watch was to simply open the Yellow Pages and evaluate the types of medical practices listed in the area. I found that there was not one female provider of gynecologic services in the section of town where I was planning to open! That one fact helped me develop my marketing "niche," making my practice different from the others. Besides being female, I would also be the only nurse practitioner practicing in that section of town.

Whatever type of practice you intend to open, you need a plan of action (or action plan) to convert your concept into an actual operating business. The standard practice when developing a business is to create a "business plan." This document, which is outlined later in this text, is often used to develop a venture by specifying short-term plans, long-term plans, and objectives. Once the business is underway, the business plan can be modified. This is your working "care plan." The business plan can also be used as a measuring tool for business performance. Initially, creating a business plan may seem overwhelming, but it is well worth your time. Creating a business plan forces you to consider some very important questions regarding how to run a successful business.

Just as you listed your personal goals, strengths, and weaknesses on the two worksheets, you should also list the strengths and weaknesses of your proposed business. In short, you should research your business ideas and determine whether they mesh with your personality and background. You should look at your skills, interests, and personal qualities objectively. In looking at your strengths and weaknesses, you should seriously plan ways to overcome challenges before you start your new venture. All of these preparations will help you determine whether you are ready to assume the role of business owner. In addition, they may reshape your ideas in planning the management of your office.

Once you have defined your practice on paper, answer the following series of questions. Your answers will help you make early decisions on whether you are ready to start a practice.

Do you have the skills needed to run the business of the practice?

Do you know what help you will need and where to find that help?

Do you have the time to learn what you may need to know?

Can you afford to hire staff or pay consultants?

Are you genuinely interested in opening this business?

Are you committed to the success of this business?

Are you willing to devote the time needed to develop this business?

Is there sufficient local demand for your services?

Can you effectively compete in the marketplace with your idea?

Will you understand your business financial statements?

Have you started to develop a business plan?

CREATING YOUR NICHE

One of the most important questions to ask yourself while planning your practice is "What will make my practice different or special?" This is such an individual thing, and it depends on the type of practice you plan to open as well as your community and competition. Get ready for the question "Why should I come to you instead of my regular doctor?" Prepare a statement including the appropriate responses, such as:

- You will receive high-quality, affordable health care.
- You may be seen on the same day that you call.
- You will not have a long wait once you arrive.
- You will be treated with respect.
- I will listen to all of your concerns.
- I have friendly staff.

- I have a nice clean office.
- My office is close by.
- Plus, I charge half of what the doctors across the street charge!

Take a moment and really think about what you have to offer and write it down. This may help when you start planning your advertising strategies.

If you are planning to start a unique or nontraditional practice, you need to investigate how you will be paid. Many nurse practitioners would like to open practices using terms such as *holistic, preventive, health maintenance,* and *consulting,* but the big question is "How will you be paid?" It is great to have altruistic thoughts, but you must be realistic. You will have bills to pay. You may want to consider starting with a more traditional practice while including some of your alternative services. Over time, you can evaluate whether you can steer your practice toward your original concept. While thinking along these terms, you may want to think about the difference between being an idealist and being a realist. Ideally, it would be awesome to provide free health care for all; realistically, you cannot run a business without charging for your services.

ESTABLISHING A PLAN OF ACTION

The development of your own practice should be taken one step at a time. Those steps are to:

1. Establish personal and business goals.
2. Investigate the viability of your business.
3. Make key decisions based on research.
4. Convert decisions into a plan of action.
5. Objectively evaluate the results of each step contributing to your plan of action.

Starting any new business requires research and careful planning. Your notion of an opportunity should be proven realistic and justified with the fact that there is a genuine need for the services you wish to provide.

Many factors and characteristics identify one business as being attractive and another as being one to avoid. These factors differ subjectively from one person to the next, being significant to one individual but not to another. Whatever type of practice you are contemplating, base your decisions on thorough, objective research. This research could involve various approaches, including marketing analysis, consumer surveys, census data reviews, and trend analysis. In short, you need to both justify and analyze the potential of your business.

Many people recommend new business developers take business courses, read texts, and consult professionals. The demands of private practice warrant that you seek all the help you possibly can, whatever the source. This holds true especially in those areas of potential value or where you have recognized a personal weakness.

One final note: Even though you may seek guidance from others, there is no substitute for the actual experience of operating an independent practice as a nurse practitioner.

THE POSITIVES OF INDEPENDENT PRACTICE

Establishing and operating your own practice has some incredible benefits. You can design the practice to be what you want it to be—the practice of your dreams! Many nurse practitioners strive to have the opportunity to practice autonomously. There is a sense of freedom that is kept in check by a feeling of responsibility. Having the ability to schedule your patients around your life is a definite benefit. There is a great sense of pride in saying "This is my practice. I own it, I run it, and, no, there are not any doctors working here." You get to be the key "decision maker." You decide how to pay the bills, set up the charts, schedule the patients, and much, much more. If you like to be in control—independent practice is for you.

The opportunities that arise with business ownership can be absolutely incredible. The satisfaction of providing the kind of care you intended to your patients and running your own business feels great.

Financial benefits include business write-offs that you may have never had before. Furthermore, your business can pay for certain things that you had paid for in the past. For example, instead of buying a car yourself, you may want your practice to buy or lease a vehicle. There are many possibilities, but you need to meet with your accountant to gain a clear understanding of these financial aspects of your business. The last thing you want is trouble with the Internal Revenue Service (IRS). Of course, you are planning to make a nice living with your practice. You may eventually sell your practice, so you'll want to build value into your business.

Throughout the years, I have thought that the positives of independent practice far outweigh the negatives.

NEGATIVES OF INDEPENDENT PRACTICE

To be fair, there are possible negatives of owning your own practice. With proper planning, though, you may not have to experience these negatives.

Because most businesses fail as a result of poor planning and poor capitalization, you can plan around the pitfalls.

Financial Stress   By doing your homework and thinking through potential obstacles before you reach them, you can save yourself a lot of grief and possibly a lot of money. The financial aspects of the practice can bring a great deal of stress. But, if you do your planning and keep close track of things, you will have a better chance for success.

Family Strain   There is also strain on the family life. You may find yourself devoting time to your business that you would rather give your family. You may want to sketch a tentative schedule that you believe you can work with, then share it with your family. Have an open discussion. Ask your family for their support and whether they will be able to live with your proposed schedule. If they say "Yes," then stick to the original schedule as much as possible, or have another meeting to discuss necessary changes.

Your Own Health   Most business owners wrestle with stress. You must take care of yourself if you want to take care of your patients. Institute or continue a daily exercise routine. Exercise is a great stress reliever. You may want to join a local organization of small business owners. It is comforting to be around people with similar challenges. Having friends who understand the pressures of making payroll, IRS concerns, rotten landlords, and the like, can be very helpful and comforting. It is nice to know that you are not the only one struggling with certain issues.

Responsibility   You will be responsible not only for patient care and follow-up, but also for employees, fire inspections, the leaky roof, the broken air conditioner, collections, payments due, and taxes. Oh! So much fun! (It really is, you just have to take it all on like a sport!)

I'll say it again, I truly believe that the benefits far outweigh the negatives of establishing and operating an independent practice.

SUGGESTIONS AND TIPS FROM WOMEN'S HEALTH WATCH, INC.

- Some practitioners may not feel comfortable working in an office as the sole practitioner. That is okay. What is most important is to recognize your strengths and weaknesses before committing yourself to independent practice.

- If you are contemplating private practice, you must assess your ability to deal with stress. One way I have kept stress under control is by exchanging the word "problem" with the word "challenge." It is much more fun to deal with a "challenge" than a "problem" or even a "crisis."

■ The final decision on making the commitment to start your own practice should be yours and yours alone. Do not do it for someone else. And, if you really don't want to commit, then don't. The sacrifice will be yours.

■ With the health-care delivery system undergoing major changes on a daily basis, evaluate your potential practice thoroughly before making the commitment. Is managed care big in your community? Do they pay independent nurse practitioners? How about Medicaid? Do they allow Nurse Practitioners to be on their provider panel? What are the limitations?

■ Some of my best "advisors" were friends and family. They were instrumental in creating the name of my practice. You may have a friend or family member who has experience with marketing, bookkeeping, or legal issues. Arrange for them to work with you if possible.

■ If you are still interested in independent practice, it is now time to set up a binder with dividers. Make sections labeled *Office Supplies*, *Medical Supplies*, *Licenses*, *Office Space*, *Patient Payments*, and so on. Write down everything you need to purchase or learn about in the different sections.

PERSONAL ANECDOTES

1. One of the personal weaknesses I identified while developing my practice is that I really do not like talking about money. Whether it is to my family, friends, employees, patients, and even to my accountant! It just makes me uncomfortable. So, I learned to work around it. By sharing my "weakness," we have been able to laugh about it and handle things in a way that I am comfortable with. My office manager handles all of the financial conversations with patients and some of our business contacts. My certified public accountant even laughs with me when we have to meet and I keep stalling. She knows I don't want to talk about my finances. She says she thinks I would be more comfortable going for a gynecological exam than talking about my financial reports. You know, I think she is right!

2. When I was trying to figure out why my patients were traveling so far to come to see me at my office I was stumped. Maybe I was guilty of low self-esteem, but I just couldn't understand why several of my patients would ride a bus over an hour to come for an appointment. I know there are health-care providers in their community. My curiosity

got the best of me, and I had to ask. I was so pleased with the responses I received. Some of them include:

- "The lady that answered the phone was so nice and patient with me."
- "You really listen when I tell you what is bothering me."
- "Seeing a woman for my female problems is very important to me."
- "You are always so nice to me."
- "You have small hands!" (I guess that was what was important to this elderly lady coming for her gynecological exam!)

3. When I was wondering and worrying whether I would be able to build a successful practice and make a profit, I sat down with paper and pen and added up all of my figures, estimating the total amount I could lose in a year. When I totaled the amount, I had to laugh, I have three older brothers, each of whom owed me more than what I thought I could lose in a year! I decided to take the risk, and if I failed, I would just take it that I had another brother!

NOTES

Chapter 2

The Professional Nurse Practitioner: Am I Really Ready?

" Hold yourself for a higher standard than anybody else expects of you "

Henry Ward Beecher

M any factors contribute to being a true professional and presenting a professional appearance to the community. This is one area you may want to assess in yourself before embarking on independent practice. Even though some of the aspects identified in this chapter may seem simple, the fact remains that making yourself into a well-rounded professional with professional behavior and appearance can make the difference between success and failure in independent practice. This chapter helps you identify aspects of your professional appearance and behavior that need to be refined before you present yourself to the community as an independent practitioner and business owner.

PROFESSIONALISM DEFINED

There are two main attributes to any profession—one is *structural* and the other is *attitudinal*. These two attributes distinguish one profession from another. Included in the structural attributes are the following:

- Formal education
- Entrance requirements
- Skill development
- Certification examination
- Licensing

The attitudinal component, or behavioral orientation, is labeled professionalism. This component conditions how individuals think about their occupation. The distinction between professionals and their professionalism is important. *Members of a profession* are determined objectively by the structural attributes listed above; *professionalism* is more individual, more subjective, and more personal. The level of professionalism reflects the practitioners' actions, behaviors, and perceptions of their work as defined by their profession.[1]

PROFESSIONAL PRESENCE

One's appearance, behavior, and speech have a direct impact on whether that person is perceived as being professional. Remember the saying, "The first impression is a lasting impression?" It is true. You want to be remembered in the best way possible, so put your best self out there every single day. Make sure your clothing is clean, wrinkle-free, and in good repair. Shoes are shined and look good. Casual dress is not for us. Your patients are paying to see a professional—look the part! If you are in wrinkled scrubs and tennis shoes they will probably think you are the office nurse or assistant. Ladies, check your makeup; less is best in this area. Too much makeup can be distracting. You want to be remembered for your excellent patient care and kindness, not your makeup. Fingernails should be clean and well maintained. Proper undergarments (you know what I am referring to!) are important too. Make sure you have a full-length mirror at home. Take a good look at yourself before you walk out the door—Is this how you want to be remembered? I know it sounds silly, but these little things add up. Patients notice details. One patient said to me "Your fingernails always look so nice and clean!" I was a surprised by the comment, but it confirmed my thoughts on good grooming.

We have all heard of people who behave "unprofessionally." Don't let it be you. Think before you speak. Think before you do anything that would reflect poorly on you, your practice, your profession, and your reputation. Never take advantage of your patients—emotionally, sexually, or financially. Public displays of inappropriate behavior (kissing on bar stools, drunkenness, cursing) may haunt you. Someone in the crowd may recognize you and that person may be or may know someone who is very important in your career success. The basic definition of the word *unprofessional* is violating the code of ethics of a given profession. Think before you act.

Professional speech encompasses gearing your conversation to the level of the listener. Never be too rushed to be polite. As harried as the workplace and pace of life can get, there is always time to be polite. Slow down; nothing can be that important. And, no matter how busy things get, put manners first, be a good listener, and always give your patients and colleagues the respect they deserve. Communication skills are divided between verbal and nonverbal. It is amazing how much you communicate without even opening your mouth! You may think you have a "poker face" and that no one can tell what you're thinking, but you may be wrong. Ask a friend whether your thoughts are readable from your expressions.

The following lists can be used to help you assess your own verbal and nonverbal communication skills.

ATTENTIVE	INATTENTIVE
Open gestures	Folding arms over chest
Eye contact	No eye contact
Nodding head	Shaking head
Commenting and restating	Sighs
Keep medical record chart open	Opening and closing chart
Aware of personal space	Touching without warning
Sitting	Side conversations
Sit, lean forward	Standing/pacing
Open-ended questions	Looking at watch
Positive voice	Rapid, loud speech

If you keep in mind the following suggestions, you can be more open and communicative with patients:

- Introduce yourself to all patients.
- Wear a name tag with title.
- Pay attention to nonverbal behaviors.
- Avoid medical jargon.
- Do not criticize others' performance.
- NEVER guarantee an outcome.
- Treat all patients courteously and with respect.
- Be considerate of their time, comfort, and privacy.
- Return calls as soon as possible.
- Present a professional image and provide patients with a positive environment.
- Address complaints and concerns.

While fine-tuning your professional presence, remember, sometimes it is the little details that make the statement. You are a professional!

DEVELOPING A RESUME OR CURRICULUM VITAE

Once you begin independent practice, it may be surprising how many times you are asked for your resume or curriculum vitae (CV). The resume is a one-to two-page summary of your employment experience. There are several standard formats. It is preferable to use the chronological format, which is outlined below. The organization of the resume can be adapted to emphasize an individual's most outstanding characteristics. In general, the resume should include:

- Identification Data: Name, address, telephone number, fax, and e-mail address.
- Objective: A single phrase expressing the specific type of employment you are seeking or the principal skills you want to use on the job. (This is really for those seeking employment—it can be omitted if you are using it for other purposes).
- Education: Basic details about your education, including college location (city and state), degree, date of graduation (or expected graduation), major, related course work, and (possibly) grade point average. Most college students do not need to include information about secondary school, but it is important to summarize education attained through community colleges, other colleges, and specialized training programs.
- Licensures: Titles and the states in which you hold licenses.
- Certification: Titles and certifying agencies.
- Employment: Brief summaries of principal employment to date. Start with your current (or most recent) position and work backward. Provide the name of the employer, the employer's address, telephone number, contact person, your job title, dates of employment, and simple phrases to summarize your main duties.
- Activities/Honors/Special Skills: Additional areas that may be included on the resume if space allows. List all major activities and awards as well as any skills that are relevant to your career objective.

Personal data such as height, weight, gender, and marital status should not be listed on the resume. Keep the resume to one or two pages (Fig. 2-1). There are businesses that can help you create or fine-tune your resume, and there are many books on preparing resumes that may give you ideas on ways to highlight your talents.

The CV is used in place of a resume for those working in academia and the sciences. The components of the CV should include the same information listed as for the resume, with the following added sections, if appropriate:

- Publications: Number in order of date of publication, put the author(s) name, the title of your publication, name of publisher, location, and date.
- Presentations: Number in order of date of presentation, put the speaker(s) name, title of presentation, location, and date.

Figure 2-1 Sample Resume.

YOUR NAME
STREET ADDRESS
CITY, STATE, ZIP CODE
TELEPHONE NUMBER
FAX NUMBER
E-MAIL ADDRESS

Objective:	To obtain a part-time associate faculty position within a nurse practitioner university program.
Education:	Broward Community College, Ft. Lauderdale, Florida 1986–1987
	Miami-Dade Community College, Miami, Florida 1987–1989: Associate's degree in nursing
	Florida International University, Miami, Florida 1989–1990: Bachelor's degree in nursing, summa cum laude
	Florida International University, Miami, Florida 1991–1992: Advanced registered nurse practitioner certificate, summa cum laude, class president
	Florida International University, Miami, Florida 1992–1993: Master's degree in nursing, clinical nurse specialist in women's health May 3, 1993, summa cum laude, charter graduate of master's program
	THESIS: "Chlamydia: Women's Knowledge and Attitudes of this Sexually Transmitted Disease"
Licensures:	Registered Nurse, State of Florida Board of Nursing
	Registered Nurse, State of New Jersey Board of Nursing
	Registered Nurse, State of Montana Board of Nursing
	Advanced Registered Nurse Practitioner, State of Florida Board of Nursing
Certifications:	Registered Nurse Certified - Ambulatory Women's Health Care Nurse, National Certification
Employment:	*Women's Health Watch, Inc.*
	4540 N. Federal Highway
	Fort Lauderdale, FL 33308
	Telephone Number
	Contact: Supervisor's Name and Title
	Duties: Independent practice of medical gynecology.
	Annual exams, family planning and general gynecological care.
	Protocol and consultations with Physician's Name, MD.

Nurse Practitioner Network
4540 N. Federal Highway
Fort Lauderdale, FL 33308
Telephone Number
Supervisor's Name and Title
Duties: Compile nurse practitioner database for use in education, marketing, and negotiations with HMOs/insurance companies.
Create monthly listing of employment opportunities within the state of Florida.

Florida Atlantic University
College of Nursing, Graduate Program
777 Glades Road
Boca Raton, FL 33431-0991
Telephone Number
Contact: Supervisor's Name and Title
Duties: Adjunct Associate Professor – Master of Nursing, Advanced Registered Nurse Practitioner Program

Florida International University
College of Nursing, Undergraduate Program
3000 NE 151st St.
N. Miami, FL 33181-3000
Telephone Number
Contact: Supervisor's Name and Title
Duties: Adjunct Associate Professor – RN to BSN transition program, Leadership Development

Broward Community College
Davie, FL
Duties: Adjunct Associate Professor – Continuing educational programs for nurses

- Research Experience: List the year of the study, the title of the study, and the institution that administered the research study.
- Special Awards: List any special awards given to you or given in your honor.[2] (Fig. 2–2).

Which is right for you? It's easy, if you have a number of presentations and publications, a CV is most appropriate for you. For everyone else, a simple one- to two-page resume is more appropriate. It is important to have an accurate, updated, and professional-appearing resume or CV (on quality paper with clear print!) to present upon request.

SCOPE OF PRACTICE

The definition of "scope of practice" for nurse practitioners varies from state to state. It is in your best interest to investigate the definition of the scope of practice for the state where you practice. Some definitions are vague and some are very clear. Specific functions that are common among many state definitions of scope of practice include the nurse practitioner's ability to:

- Diagnose
- Prescribe
- Treat
- Admit to hospital
- Repair lacerations
- Refer
- Teach
- Order tests
- Conduct advanced nursing acts

Many states require that the areas listed here be addressed in written protocols that are agreed upon by the collaborating or supervising physician and the nurse practitioner.

Learn the law, know the law, and practice within the law. Never cross that imaginary line in practice that will put your patient, yourself, and your collaborating physician in jeopardy. Perform at your level of training. Know when to refer and do it. You are not doing anyone any favors by practicing outside your scope of knowledge.

The American Academy of Nurse Practitioners has created the following definition of the scope of practice for nurse practitioners:

> *Nurse practitioners are primary care providers who practice in ambulatory acute and long-term care settings. According to their practice specialty, these primary care providers provide nursing and medical services to individuals, families, and groups. In addition to diagnosing and managing*

Figure 2-2	Sample Curriculum Vitae

CURRICULUM VITAE

NAME:	Your Name, Degrees
ADDRESS:	Business Name
	Business Address
	City, State, Zip Code
	Telephone Number
	Fax Number
	E-mail Address
Place of Birth:	Anaheim, California
Date of Birth:	February 15, 1960
Education:	Germantown High School, Germantown, Tennessee 1975–1977
	Sea Isle Vocational School, Memphis, Tennessee 1978–1979 (Surgical Technologist)
	Broward Community College, Ft. Lauderdale, Florida 1986–1987
	Miami-Dade Community College, Miami, Florida 1987–1990: Associate's degree in nursing
	Florida International University, Miami, Florida 1989–1990: Bachelor's degree in nursing, summa cum laude
	Florida International University, Miami, Florida 1991–1992: Advanced registered nurse practitioner certificate, summa cum laude, class president
	Florida International University, Miami, Florida 1992–1994: Master's degree in nursing, clinical nurse specialist in women's health May 3, 1993, summa cum laude, charter graduate of master's program
	THESIS: "Chlamydia: Women's Knowledge and Attitudes of this Sexually Transmitted Disease"
Licensures:	Registered Nurse, State of Florida Board of Nursing
	Registered Nurse, State of New Jersey Board of Nursing
	Registered Nurse, State of Montana Board of Nursing
	Advanced Registered Nurse Practitioner, State of Florida Board of Nursing
Certifications:	Registered Nurse Certified – Ambulatory Women's Health Care Nurse, National Certification
Employment:	*Women's Health Watch, Inc.*
	4540 N. Federal Highway
	Fort Lauderdale, FL 33308
	Telephone Number
	Contact: Supervisor's Name and Title
	Duties: Independent practice of medical gynecology.
	Annual exams, family planning and general gynecological care.
	Protocol and consultations with Physician's Name, MD.
	Nurse Practitioner Network
	4540 N. Federal Highway
	Fort Lauderdale, FL 33308
	Telephone Number
	Contact: Supervisor's Name and Title
	Duties: Compile nurse practitioner database for use in education, marketing, and negotiations with HMOs/insurance companies.
	Create monthly listing of employment opportunities within the state of Florida.
	Florida Atlantic University
	College of Nursing, Graduate Program
	777 Glades Road
	Boca Raton, FL 33431-0991
	Telephone Number
	Contact: Supervisor's Name and Title
	Duties: Adjunct Associate Professor – Master of Nursing, Advanced Registered Nurse Practitioner Program
	Florida International University
	College of Nursing, Undergraduate Program
	3000 NE 151st St
	N. Miami, FL 33181-3000
	Telephone Number

[Continued]

Figure 2-2 **Sample Curriculum Vitae** *[Continued]*

Contact: Supervisor's Name and Title
Duties: Adjunct Associate Professor – RN to BSN transition program, leadership development

Broward Community College
Davie, FL
Duties: Adjunct Associate Professor – Continuing educational programs for nurses

Scientific Societies and Other:
- The Honor Society of Phi Kappa Phi at Florida International University
- American Academy of Nurse Practitioners
- Association of Operating Room Nurses
- American Society of Laser Medicine and Surgery
- American Nurses Association
- Florida Nurses Association
- Debra Levy Neimark Scholarship Foundation Board
- National Association of Nurse Practitioners in Reproductive Health
- South Florida Council of Advanced Practice Nurses
- National Association of Women Business Owners (community affairs chair, 1994; secretary, 1995; vice president, 1996; VISTA chair, 1996; president, 1997; VISTA Chair, 1997; National Board representative, 1998; VISTA Chair, 1998)
- Community Liaison Governing Board Florida Atlantic University School of Nursing Graduate Program
- Women's Healthcare Executive Network
- American College of Nurse Practitioners

Publications:
1. Last Name, First Initial *Enfermedades de Transmision sexual: Una Epidemic* ("Sexually Transmitted Diseases: An Epidemic"), *La Republica Newspaper,* Bogota, Colombia, South America, January 1993.
2. Last Name, First Initial *Norplant: Una Alternativa Unica en el Control de la Natalidad* ("Norplant: A Unique Alternative in Birth Control"), *La Republica Newspaper,* Bogota, Colombia, South America, January 1993.
3. Last Name, First Initial *Terapia Con Remplazameniento Hormonal* (Hormone Replacement Therapy: Making Informed Choices"), *La Republica Newspaper,* Bogota, Colombia, South America, March 1993.
4. Last Name, First Initial *Clamidia* (Chlamydia), *La Republica Newspaper,* Bogota, Colombia, South America, April 1993.
5. Last Name, First Initial *La Endometriosis* ("Endometriosis"), *La Republica Newspaper,* Bogota, Colombia, South America, May 1993.
6. Last Name, First Initial *Cancer del Endometrio* ("Endometrial Cancer"), *La Republica Newspaper,* Bogota, Colombia, South America, May 1993.
7. Last Name, First Initial *El Juego del Ejercicio en el Control de la Obedidad* ("The Critical Role of Exercise in Weight Control"), *La Republica Newspaper,* Bogota, Colombia, South America, June 1993.
8. Last Name, First Initial *Herpes Genital* ("Herpes Simplex II"), *La Republica Newspaper,* Bogota, Colombia, South America, June 1993.

Presentations:
1. Last Name, First Initial *Chlamydia: Women's Knowledge and Attitudes of this Sexually Transmitted Disease,* Florida Nurses Association, 82nd Annual Convention, Orlando, Florida, August 23, 1993.
2. Last Name, First Initial *Chlamydia and Other STD's,* Radio Interview/Robbie George, WMXJ 102.7 FM, January 9, 1994.
3. Last Name, First Initial *Introduction to Women's Health,* Deerfield Beach High School, Deerfield Beach, FL, March 16, 1994.
4. Last Name, First Initial *Sexually Transmitted Diseases,* Radio Interview/Leo Vela, Power 96 WPOW FM, March 20, 1994.
5. Last Name, First Initial *Introduction to Women's Health,* Career City College, Fort Lauderdale, April 27, 1994.
6. Last Name, First Initial *Chlamydia: Women's Knowledge and Attitudes of this Sexually Transmitted Disease* The First International and interdisciplinary Health Research Symposium, Peking Union Medical College, Beijing, China, May 18–25, 1994.
7. Last Name, First Initial *Chlamydia: Women's Knowledge and Attitudes of this Sexually Transmitted Disease,* 1994 National Conference of the American Academy of Nurse Practitioners, Washington, DC, June 8–12, 1994.

| **Figure 2–2** | Sample Curriculum Vitae *[Continued]* |

8. Last Name, First Initial *Introduction to Women's Health,* Pine Crest Preparatory School, Fort Lauderdale, FL, May 10, 1994.
9. Last Name, First Initial *Breast Health Awareness—Mid Life Passage: Menopause*, NAWBO Health Fair, Fort Lauderdale, FL, July 11, 1994.
10. Last Name, First Initial *Introduction to Women's Health*, Bauder Collge, Fort Lauderdale, July 12, 1994.
11. Last Name, First Initial *How to Present a Thesis*, Florida International University, Miami, FL, July 28, 1994.
12. Last Name, First Initial *The Nurse Practitioner as Entrepreneur: How to Establish and Operate an Independent Practice*, Mt. Sinai Hospital, Miami Beach, FL, November 1, 1994.
13. Last Name, First Initial *The Nurse Practitioner as Entrepreneur: How to Establish and Operate an Independent Practice*, South Florida Nurse Educators, North Ridge Hospital, Fort Lauderdale, FL, March 15, 1995.
14. Last Name, First Initial *The Nurse Practitioner as Entrepreneur: How to Establish and Operate an Independent Practice*, Florida International University, Aventura Hospital, Aventura, FL, April 4, 1995.
15. Last Name, First Initial *Women's Health Issues*, Hadassah Nurses Council, Boca Raton, FL, April 5, 1995.

Research Experience:

1987–1988   Research Assistant, University of Miami, Division of Transplantation (Liver, Heart, Kidney, and Pancreas).

1993 "Chlamydia: Women's Knowledge and Attitudes of this Sexually Transmitted Disease," Florida International University – Masters Thesis.

1996–1998 QC Products, Inc., Ft. Lauderdale, FL   *Sub-Investigator:*

1. Sexually Transmitted Disease Project
2. Hepatitis A Vaccine Project: Smith-Kline & Merck
3. Sexually Transmitted Disease – Longitudinal
4. Vulvo-vaginitis Candidiasis Project

1998–1999 Millennium Biotech, Inc.   *Sub-Investigator:*

1. Hemolyzed and normal serum sample collection
2. Benign Breast Disease Study
3. Benign Gynecological Disease Study

1998–1999 Clinical Studies, Ft. Lauderdale   *Sub-Investigator:*

1. A Multicenter, double-blind, controlled randomized study to determine efficacy in the relief of hot flushes in women receiving transdermal XXX compared to oral XXX XXX
2. Continuous oral XXX XXX combinations and continuous oral XXX, examining the effect of the endometrium, symptoms, and bleeding Patterns in post menopausal women
3. A double-blind, randomized, parallel study comparing XXX XXXTD 7-day patch xx,xx, and xx μg/day with placebo in the treatment of vasomotor symptoms in postmenopausal women
4. A randomized, double-blind, active and placebo controlled, parallel group multicenter study assessing the safety and protective effect on the endometrium of XXX dosage combinations of XXX XXX plus XXX XXX.

Special Presentations:

Name of Research Award at Florida International University presented to:

• Name mo/yr   • Name mo/yr   • Name mo/yr

Special Awards:

• South Florida Council of Advanced Nurse Practitioners • 1995 Nurse Practitioner of the Year Florida Nurses Association/Broward County • 1995 Nurse of the Year Finalist • NAWBO Member of the Year 1995 • Finalist VISTA Awards • Certificate of Recognition as 1st Vice President Board of Directors South Florida Council of Advanced Nurse Practitioners • Florida Nurses Association Council on Advanced Nursing Practice 1995 PEARL Award • Certificate of Merit Award 1995 American Academy of Nurse Practitioners • Price Waterhouse Up & Comers Award Finalist 1995 • National Association of Women Business Owner of the Year Broward County 1996 NAWBO Nominee • *Women's Business Journal* July 1996 Woman of the Month • Price Waterhouse Up & Comers Award 1997 Winner/Healthcare Division • National Association of Women Business Owners 1999 VISTA Winner (Vision in Service to Associations) • Named *"One of the 10 Most Powerful Women in Broward County" Women's Business Journal*, November 12, 1999 *acute episodic and chronic illnesses, nurse practitioners emphasize health promotion and disease prevention. Service includes but is not limited to ordering, conducting, and interpreting diagnostic and laboratory tests, prescription of pharmacologic agents, and treatments and nonpharmacologic therapies. Teaching and counseling individuals, families, and groups are a major part of nurse practitioner's practice. Nurse practitioners practice autonomously and in collaboration with health-care professionals and other individuals to diagnose, treat, and manage the patient's health problems. They serve as health-care resources, interdisciplinary consultants, and patient advocates.[3]*

Other associations may have developed their own definitions of the scope of practice for the nurse practitioner. Many believe that the Board of Nursing keeps a list of acceptable and unacceptable tasks and procedures that nurse practitioners are allowed to perform. This is not the case. With changes in medical procedures happening almost daily, making such a list of acceptable tasks would not be practical. Typically, when a scope of practice question is raised, the determination is based upon what knowledge and skills are necessary for the safe completion of the task and what potential complications may arise. Many tasks require advanced training and experience. Once the nurse practitioner has mastered the task or procedure and maintains proficiency, the task may be safely accomplished within that nurse practitioner's scope of practice. If a task or procedure has potential complications, the nurse practitioner must be able to intervene to protect the client from further harm if such a complication occurs. Your Board of Nursing or licensing body can provide a current definition of the nurse practitioner's scope of practice for your state.

CONTINUING EDUCATION

Keeping current with the research and changes in medicine is our duty as nurse practitioners. Many states require that a certain number of Continuing Education Units (CEUs) be acquired over a certain period of time. Certifying bodies for national certification also may require a certain number of continuing education contact hours over a certain time frame. Your nursing board or licensing body can give you the state requirements. Certifying agencies also state the continuing education requirements in their literature.

There are many different ways to attain continuing education credits, including authoring journal articles, attending nurse practitioner meetings, taking college courses, and participating in educational programs and Internet programs. Your state may require specific courses be taken for continued licensure, such as courses on domestic violence, child abuse, or HIV updates. Know the requirements and complete the required work. If you don't, you could lose your license! Constantly reading and updating your knowledge base will keep you on the cutting edge of research development, which is of significant benefit to you and your patients.

NATIONAL CERTIFICATION

Many states now require National Certification for licensure of nurse practitioners; whereas, in the past, this was considered optional. The national certifying agencies include the American Academy of Nurse Practitioners, American Nurses Credentialing Center, National Certification Board of Pediatric Nurse Practitioners, and Nurses and the National Certification Corporation. To become certified, you must pass an examination administered by one of these agencies. Then, you must adhere to their specific continuing education requirements and pay dues. There are many benefits to attaining and maintaining national certification. Certification provides evidence to the client and the community that the individual has achieved knowledge beyond basic nursing. Studies have shown that national certification has a dramatic impact on personal, professional, and practice outcomes of certified nurses, and it is a key tool in reducing health-care errors. Studies have also shown that nationally certified nurses had high patient satisfaction ratings, that they had more effective communication and collaboration with other health-care providers, and that they experienced fewer adverse events and errors in patient care than before they were certified. Nationally certified nurse practitioners reported feeling more confident in their abilities to detect early signs and symptoms of complications and to initiate early and prompt interventions.[4] See Table 2–1 for the certifying agencies and their contact information. Review courses for the different specialties and their contact information are listed in Table 2–2.

SERVING AS A MENTOR OR PRECEPTOR

Mentors have been described as role models and guides who encourage and inspire. Other descriptions include teacher, advocate, counselor, and confidante. Being a mentor can be rewarding for the nurse practitioner, but it can also be frustrating and exhausting. Mentoring requires a high degree of commitment, involvement, and energy. Mentoring is a mutual process of transformation, one that inspires and enriches lives.

The nurse practitioner in independent practice may be torn when asked to serve as a preceptor or mentor to nurse practitioner students. Especially during the first few years of developing your business, you will have to evaluate whether you can afford to donate your time to a student.

If you do decide to venture into the preceptor/mentor role, there are several things to keep in mind that will help make the experience more meaningful for you and the student. You should insist on an orientation from the requesting university. Learn exactly what is expected from you and learn the time frame. Set goals with the student, and define specific skills or experiences they need to learn. As a preceptor, you will be sharing your expert clinical knowledge base, assisting the student in gaining confidence as a provider, and sharing the role of the nurse practitioner with the student.

Table 2-1 Certifying Agencies	
American Academy of Nurse Practitioners (AANP) P.O. Box 12846 Austin, TX 78711 512-442-4262 *admin@aanp.org; www.aanp.org*	Adult Family
American Nurses Credentialing Center (ANCC) 600 Maryland Ave., SW, #100W Washington, DC 20024-2571 1-800-284-2378 *ancc@ana.org; www.nursingworld.org/ancc*	Adult Family Pediatric Geriatric Acute care School nurse practioner
National Certification Board of Pediatric Nurse Practitioners & Nurses 800 S. Frederick Ave., Suite 104 Gaithersburg, MD 20877-4150 301-330-2921 *info@pnpcert.org; www.pnpcert.org*	Pediatric (NCBNP/N)
National Certification Corporation (NCC) P.O. Box 11082 Chicago, IL 60611 312-951-0207 *www.nccnet.org*	Women's Health Care Neonatal
ACNM Certification Council Inc. (ACC) 8401 Corporate Drive, Suite 630 Landover, MD 20785 301-459-1321 *acnmcertcn@aol.com*	Midwifery

Table 2-2 Providers of Certification Review Courses	
Fitzgerald Health Education Associates, Inc. 11 Appletree Lane Andover, MA 01810-4101 1-800-927-5380 *www.fhea.com*	Adult Family Geriatric Women's Health
Advanced Practice Education Associates 103 Darwin Circle Lafayette, LA 70508 *Infor@apea.com; www.apea.com* 1-800-899-4502	Adult Family
Health Leadership Associates, Inc. P.O. Box 59153 Potomac, MD 20859 1-800-435-4775 *www.healthleadership.com*	Adult Family Gerontological Women's Health Acute Care Pediatric Midwifery
Towson's Educational Enterprises/Entities P.O. Box 20374 Towson, MD 21284 1-800-225-6506 *www.necessarynp.com*	Adult Family Geriatric

NURSE PRACTITIONER ORGANIZATIONS

The benefits of becoming active in nurse practitioner organizations can be invaluable. You can network, learn, and grow your practice with the knowledge and connections gained from your association.

The first place to start is locally. Is there a nurse practitioner group within your community? Maybe there is an organization within your county or region. The next question is whether or not there is a state nurse practitioner organization. And, of course, there are several national nurse practitioner organizations.

Each level of organization has specific member benefits. The community or county group addresses issues that are specific to your local area, whereas the national associations work for all nurse practitioners in many different ways. They help define the scope of practice of the nurse practitioners, address concerns of nurse practitioners, provide conferences, provide continuing education programs, administer certifying examinations, give legislative updates, and even lobby for legislative changes that benefit nurse practitioners. It is suggested that you investigate and get involved in all levels of nurse practitioner associations. Table 2–3 lists national nurse practitioner organizations and their contact information.

NURSE PRACTITIONER JOURNALS

The information contained in nurse practitioner journals is invaluable. Journals contain recent research, continuing education articles, job advertisements, new products, legislative changes, and many other topics of interest. Some of the journals are given free with certain association memberships. Table 2–4 lists nurse practitioner journals and their contact information. I have included one that is not a nurse practitioner journal that could be beneficial to the nurse practitioner in independent practice. That journal is *Medical Economics*, which contains articles that have to do with practice management and other issues for independent practitioners. There are many other magazines that are focused on small business. You will want to try to keep current and learn more about the business of the practice.

SUGGESTIONS AND TIPS FROM WOMEN'S HEALTH WATCH, INC.

■ Instituting a dress code before you open your practice may save you a lot of headaches later on. My office manager either wore a dress or nice pants with a coordinating blouse. I always wore a dress or a skirt and blouse. I wore a white lab coat with my name embroidered above the pocket. We never wore blue jeans, scrubs, or athletic shoes.

Table 2-3 National Nurse Practitioner Organizations

American Academy of Nurse Practitioners (AANP)
P.O. Box 12846
Austin, TX 78711
512-442-4262
admin@aanp.org; www.aanp.org

American College Health Association (ACHA) Nurse/NP Sections
P.O. Box 28937
Baltimore, MD 21240-8937
410- 859-1500
aaohn@aaohn.org; www.aaohn.org

American College of Nurse-Midwives
818 Connecticut Ave. NW, Suite 900
Washington, DC 20006
202-728-9860
info@acnm.org

American College of Nurse Practitioners (ACNP)
1090 Vermont Ave. NW, Suite 800
Washington, DC 20005
202- 408-7050
acnp@nurse.org; www.nurse.org/acnp

American Nurses Association (ANA)
Council of Advanced Practice Nurses
600 Maryland Ave. SW, Suite 100 W
Washington, DC 20024-2571
202- 651-7000
doneal@ana.org; www.NursingWorld.org

Association of Advanced Practice Psychiatric Nursing
c/o Connie Huffine
5550 33rd Ave, NE
Seattle, WA 98105
206-524-4090
chfox@u.washington.edu

National Alliance of Nurse Practitioners
325 Pennsylvania Ave., SE
Washington, DC 20003
202-675-6350

National Association Nurse Practitioners in Reproductive Health (NANPRH)
1090 Vermont Ave., NW #800
Washington, DC 20005
202-408-7025
nanprh@nurse.org; www.nurse.org/nanprh

National Association of Pediatric Nurse Associates and Practitioners (NAPNAP)
1101 Kings Hwy. N, #206
Cherry Hill, NJ 08034-1912
609-667-1773
74224.51@compuserve.com; www.napnap.org

National Conference of Gerontological Nurse Practitioners (NCGNP)
P.O. Box 270101
Fort Collins, CO 80527-0101
970-493-7793
ncgnp@frii.com

National Organization of Nurse Practitioner Faculties (NONPF)
One Dupont Circle NW, Suite 530
Washington, DC 20036
202-452-1405
nonpf@aacn.nche.edu

Nurse Practitioner Associates for Continuing Education (NPACE)
5 Militia Drive
Lexington, MA 02173
617-861-0270
npace@npace.com

Uniformed Nurse Practitioner Association (UNPA)
Health Care Resources
1153 Bergen Pkwy., M181
Evergreen, CO 80439
1-800-759-2881
m2hra@aol.com

Table 2-4	Nurse Practitioner Journals

Advance for Nurse Practitioners
Merion Publications, Inc.
650 Park Ave.
King of Prussia, PA 19406-0956
1-800-355-1088

American Journal for Nurse Practitioners
800 Business Center Drive, Suite 100
Horsham, PA 19044

American Journal of Nursing
P.O. Box 50480
Boulder, CO 80322-0480
1-800-627-0484
www.nursingcenter.com/subscribe

APNSCAN
Paymark Communications, Inc.
33 Main Street
Old Saybrook, CT 06475-9896
860-395-0512

The Clinical Advisor for Nurse Practitioners
7 Skyline Drive
Hawthorne, NY 10532-2179
914-347-3800
subscriptions@clinicaladvisor.com

Clinical Excellence for Nurse Practitioners
Periodicals Department
WB Saunders
6277 Sea Harbor Drive
Orlando, FL 32887-4800
1-800-654-2452

Clinical Letter for Nurse Practitioners
P.O. Box 23291
Baltimore, MD 21203-9990
1-800-638-6423
custserv@wwilkins.com

Clinician News
Clinicians Publishing Group
Two Brighton Road, Suite 300
Clifton, NY 07012
973-916-1000

Clinician Reviews
Clinician Publishing Group
Two Brighton Road, Suite 300
Clifton, NY 07012
973-916-1000
clinrev@clinicianspublishing.com

Consultant
55 Holly Hill Lane
Box 4010
Greenwich, CT 06831-0010

Journal of the American Academy of Nurse Practitioners
Capitol Station, LBJ Building
P.O. Box 12846
Austin, TX 78711

Medical Economics
Medical Economics Subscriber Services Department
P.O. Box 3000
Denville, NJ 07834-9662
1-800-432-4570

[Continued]

Table 2–4	Nurse Practitioner Journals *[Continued]*

Nurse Practitioner Journal
P.O. Box 5053
Brentwood, TN 37024-5053
1-800-490-6580

Nurse Practitioner World News
800 Business Center Drive, Suite 100
Horsham, PA 19044

Nurse Practitioners Prescribing Reference
Prescribing Reference, Inc.
Attn: NPSD
170 Broadway, Suite 1612
New York, NY 10007
1-800-436-9269

Patient Care Nurse Practitioner
Medical Economics, Subscriber Services Dept.
Patient Care Nurse Practitioner
P.O. Box 3000
Denville, NJ 07834-9662
1-800-432-4570

- Why should you keep your resume or CV updated when you have your own practice? I have been asked for copies of my CV by people in the media when I have been interviewed. When I speak at conferences, the organizers need a copy to keep on file for continuing education provider requirements. The universities I have been affiliated with have requested copies. It is a nice way to let people know who you are and what you have accomplished.

- Your scope of practice should change over the years as you master more skills. Be sure to log any new skills training you have completed as well as all supervised practice sessions.

PERSONAL ANECDOTES

1. I had a full-length mirror installed in the lounge of my office. I cannot count how many times it saved me from going to see patients looking unkempt. I found crumbs on my face, lipstick on my teeth, my slip hanging down, runs in my hose, and much more. Obviously, not the way I would want to be remembered!

2. After about a year of independent practice, I really wanted to learn how to perform colposcopy (an office procedure to assess cervical changes after an abnormal Pap smear). I spoke with my collaborating physician and we mapped out a plan. I completed the educational course and felt ready to share my skills with the world! I have a nurse midwife friend who was an expert colposcopist. We set up a day for colposcopies only

at her office. She was with a very large practice, so this wasn't too difficult to do. After spending the day with her, I spent a couple more days working with my collaborating physician. He then cleared me to perform colposcopies without his being present. I did them at my office and set up a logbook. I also put together a folder with a copy of the abnormal Pap, my procedure record, biopsy reports, and photos of the cervix. I made my recommendations on the procedure sheet. My physician of protocol reviewed the packages and signed his name next to my recommended plan. This way, I felt confident that I could clearly show my training as well as the supervision I had for my first 200 colposcopies. Thank goodness I never had to defend my training. It gave me great comfort to know that I had done everything possible to document my actions.

3. It's easy to become lax about continuing education credits—don't do it! I was part of a "random audit" performed by the Board of Nursing. I had to show documentation of all CEUs acquired during a certain time frame, my management protocol, and the letter to the Board of Medicine (required by Florida law). I was so nervous the day I received the letter. I called my office manager and told her I needed 20 CEUs during the time frame in the letter. She called me back to let me know there was no problem—I had 180 CEUs! I had her copy all 180 records and sent them to the Board of Nursing. Imagine the panic you might feel if you get audited and haven't completed the hours.

Resources

Ireland, S: The Complete Idiot's Guide to the Perfect Resume, 2nd ed. New York: Alpha Books, 2000.
Jackson, AL: Prepare Your Curriculum Vitae (Here's How). NTC Publishing Company, Lincolnwood, IL, 1998.
Maister, DH: True Professionalism: The Courage to Care About Your People, Your Clients, and Your Career. Touchstone Books, New York, 2000.
Peddy, S: The Art of Mentoring: Lead, Follow and Get Out of the Way. Learning Connections, New York, 1999.
http://www.nurse.net/npcentral

References

1. Lusch, RF, and O'Brien, M: Fostering professionalism. Market Res 9, 25–31, 1997.
2. Mississippi State University Cooperative Education Program, Resume Writing, at *http://www.msstate.edu/Dept/Coop/interview/resume.html.*
3. American Academy of Nurse Practitioners: *http:www.aanp.org.*
4. Peters, S: Too much information? Washington debates medical errors reporting. Am J Nurse Pract 3:30, 2000.

N O T E S

Chapter 3

Analyzing the Potential of Your Business: Can I Really Do This?

" What the mind of man can conceive and believe, the mind of man can achieve "

Napoleon Hill

Now is the time to sit down with a pen and paper and start drafting the basic design of your practice. This helps you prepare for writing your business plan and launching your practice. Let's start by defining your practice by answering the four W's: who, what, where, and when.

DEFINING YOUR PRACTICE

Who

Who will operate this practice? *Who* will own the practice? Will you be working with a partner? There are definite advantages and disadvantages with working with others. You know whether you work better on your own or with others. Think back to those "group projects" in school. Were you able to really work well with a group? Did you feel more comfortable with group projects or solo projects? Did you do all of the work for the group and let them share the good grade you received?

One of the main benefits of solo practice is the autonomy. It is all yours, the good and the bad. The financial responsibility, patient responsibility, taxes, decisions, productivity—it's all up to you! The rewards of having your own business can be awesome! You can say you did it all by yourself! If you decide you would feel more comfortable with a partner or group, you may find power in numbers. It may be easier to locate lenders for financing. You will get to share the responsibilities in the business and in patient care. Plus, you will have someone who truly understands what you are going through.

Who will be your patients? Try to identify your patient group. Define who you plan on seeing as patients. Basically, this is considered your "target market." Will it include boys and girls from birth to age 16? Will it be all women during their reproductive years? Try to nail down who your potential patients will be.

Who will be your collaborating or supervising physician (depending on your state laws)? Do you have someone in mind? Have you spoken with him or her? Is that person truly supportive of your plan or would he or she just be doing it with a "what's in it for me?" attitude? It really is nice to have someone who is truly supportive with whom you have a good rapport.

Who will you need to hire? Can you run your practice with just one employee or do you need more?

What

What type of services will you provide? Will you be selling products? *What* type of practice would you like to start? Family practice? Women's health? Pediatrics?

Where

Where will you practice? You may already have an exact address confirmed for your practice or you may still be investigating areas of town that would be best for your proposed practice. If you are trying to decide on a location, there are several ways to investigate where you should start your practice. Ask around; the sales representatives from the pharmaceutical companies know a lot about the practices in the area. They may be able to give you invaluable information. Ask other practitioners in the area. And then, address one of your most valuable tools, the Yellow Pages. Take a map of the area and make red marks at each location where your competitors have practices. You will then be able to see whether they are all located in the same area or are spread throughout the county.

The actual section of town may not be as important as the exterior of your potential office. Having a sign on a busy road in front of your practice is definitely better than being on the 8th floor of a tall building without signage.

Assess the safety of the neighborhood. Will you feel comfortable coming and going at all hours? Drive by at night—are there "undesirables" hanging around the building?

Where will your patient payments come from? Are you designing a self-pay only practice? Will you be depending on Medicare and Medicaid for payments? Insurance companies? HMOs? You don't have to decide today what percent of your patients will be Medicaid, but you do need to have an idea of where your reimbursements will be coming from. Will these payments be able to cover your office expenses?

Where will referrals come from?

When

When would you like to open your practice? This date can be changed later if you need more time or maybe you will be ready sooner than planned. Set a date, a projected date when you will be able to open your doors for patient care. You may be able to make all of the arrangements and open your doors in 3 months or you may want to take your time and open in a year or two. Do not let anyone push you to open before you are ready. You need to be confident that you have everything in order to provide quality health care.

These first decisions will set you on the road to planning a successful practice. Once you have answered the basic questions, it is time to work out the details.

ESTIMATING YOUR START-UP COSTS

This exercise is very important when attempting to analyze the financial potential of your proposed business. It may be the task that helps you decide whether or not you will be starting your own practice. Take a look at Figure 3–1 and we can go through the items one by one:

Office Space   The first decision to be made is whether you wish to have your own office or share space in an established health-care facility. There are advantages and disadvantages to both scenarios with financing playing a significant role in the outcome. Obviously, a freestanding office will initially require more funding. In addition, by sharing an office, certain expenditures and support staff could also be arranged on a shared basis. For a variety of reasons, Women's Health Watch opened in a freestanding building. In selecting an office, the most important factors are location, cost, and available space. In terms of location, a high traffic area increases visibility and, in turn, increases the likelihood of attracting more clients.

Check around in the area where you want to open your practice. If you see an office you would consider appropriate, then call the realtor and ask questions:

- What is the size of the office (square feet)?
- How much is the monthly rent?
- When is it available?
- What are the move-in costs (first month's rent, last month's rent, security deposit)?

Some of the things you should look for when you are considering a property are:

1. A building that is well maintained and in good condition.
2. An explanation of the common areas you will be able to use, with parking being a critical factor.

Figure 3-1 **Estimated Start-up Costs Worksheet.**

	Initial Costs	Monthly Costs
Office space		
First, last and security deposit		
Monthly charge		
Renovation (add counter, move walls, etc.)		
Utilities		
Water		
Garbage		
Power		
Hazardous waste disposal		
Telephone		
Office equipment		
Office maintenance and cleaning		
Pest control		
Outdoor signage		
Medical equipment		
Building and business insurance		
Security system		
Office supplies		
Medical supplies		
Licenses		
MD consulting fee		
Bank fees		
Advertising		
Printing		
Laboratory fees		
Payroll		
Payroll taxes		
Sales tax		
Professional fees		
Health insurance		
Liability insurance		
Disability insurance		
Continuing education		
Entertainment and promotions		
Auto		
Association dues		
Subscriptions		

3. The right to renew your lease when it expires.

4. A list of the building services covered by the agreement (e.g., water, garbage removal, power).

5. An understanding of rights to make any improvements.

6. Location of walls, sinks, countertops—will you need renovations?

7. An understanding of who is responsible for the maintenance of exterior property, such as mowing the lawn and trimming the hedges.

Utilities   You will want to estimate the monthly charges for the utilities that will be your responsibility and find out what deposits are required for:

- Water
- Garbage (regular and hazardous waste)
- Power

Tolophone   Again, estimate your monthly charges and determine whether any deposits are required. Check out the existing telephone equipment in your new office. Will you need to replace the current system or is it functional? Estimate the cost for implementation or installation of the following:

- Basic monthly charge (service contracts, equipment charges, taxes)
- Long distance charges
- Fax line
- Internet (Website, e-mail)
- Toll free number (if necessary)
- Telephone equipment lease or purchase (if necessary)
- Answering service
- Beeper
- Cellular telephone

Office Equipment   There are many options to consider with office equipment. Some items you may be able to lease or purchase used. You may want to opt for a service contract when you purchase your equipment. You may also be able to consolidate your equipment—for example, some computer printers also work as a fax, a scanner, and a copier. You will need the following:

- Computer and software programs (medical records, bookkeeping, and word processing programs)
- Printer
- Fax
- Copy machine

- Credit card processing terminal
- Postage machine (optional)
- Typewriter
- Coffee machine
- Water cooler rental and bottled water
- Microwave
- Small refrigerator (for employee lunches)
- Small refrigerator (for medications)
- Small refrigerator (for laboratory specimens)

Office Maintenance and Cleaning Will you need to hire a handyman to do repairs or do you have a friend or family member who can help you with maintenance? Is your office staff willing and able to do a thorough weekly cleaning? Do you need to hire a service or pay a staff member to clean the office?

Pest Control In South Florida, this is a necessity. Whatever you do for your house in this area, you should also do for your office.

Outdoor Signage In addition to having a sign on the front door, a large sign should be created and hung on the outside of your office building. The lettering on this sign should be large enough to be read from the road and should be lit throughout the night.

Medical Equipment This is definitely an area that is "practice type specific." Make a list of every piece of medical equipment you will need, from the otoscope to any other high-tech equipment you need to start practicing. Then, compare prices, both for new and used items. You may also want to check out leasing agreements for the equipment.

Building and Business Insurance Call your insurance agent and learn about the different policies available and their premiums. If you are renting your office, your insurance costs will be different than if you own it. Certain types of insurance are available to help you if your building is destroyed and you are unable to practice. Check it out and weigh it out. You can always change your insurance coverage later. Make sure that you are neither underinsured nor overinsured.

Security System There are many reasons to consider setting up a security system. Check with your neighboring businesses regarding the history of burglaries in your neighborhood. If you have expensive equipment or medications, you may become a target for burglars. Many alarm systems can record the time when the first person enters your office in the morning and the last person exits your office at night. You may even be able to program the security system to act as a time clock for employees. There is also the option for silent alarm, in case someone threatening comes through your front door. If you live in a safe little community, this may all be unnecessary.

Office Supplies   Make a list of every little thing you need to run the front office. List everything from copy paper to paperclips. This may be a long list, but be thorough. You can use this list to price shop later on.

Medical Supplies   List everything you will need to purchase to practice—tongue depressors, sutures, dressings, table paper, gowns, and so on.

Licenses   You must investigate which licenses you need to run a business in your area. City and county business licenses are standard. Biohazard waste requirements for your state need to be investigated. Of course, you will always keep your professional license current. All of these licenses have fees for application and renewal—list out the fees.

MD Consulting Fees   Depending on the arrangement with your collaborating or supervising physician, you may have to budget a payment for their services.

Bank Fees   Explore the cost for business checking. Some banks are more "small business friendly" than others. Some have programs with reduced fees, free checks, and extra services. Inquire about establishing a "line of credit" for your practice. A line of credit works like a credit card for your business. You can write checks from this account and pay it back as you can. Check the fees on this account as well.

If you are going to be accepting credit cards, you can expect an application fee, a monthly statement fee, and a small percentage fee for each transaction.

Advertising   This is a difficult area to estimate. Once you have your marketing plan in place, you will be able to project your advertising costs with more certainty. This is an area where you really need to be careful. It is very easy to spend a lot of money in a short amount of time on advertising. Plan your strategy, know the costs, and work within your budget. There are many different theories on the best ways to market your practice. It also depends on your community. Estimate approximate monthly costs for advertisements in the:

- Yellow Pages
- Newspaper
- Radio/TV

Printing   It is important to present a professional appearance, even in correspondence. Good quality printed material will be noticed and appreciated. Find a good printer who will work with you in designing a professional, but affordable, set of stationary and business cards. A graphic designer can work with you to develop a logo specific for your practice. Estimate the costs for the following printing projects:

- Logo design
- Letterhead
- Second page stationery (paper to match letterhead)
- Envelopes
- Business cards
- Appointment cards
- Brochures
- Signs for inside the office (e.g., "Exam room 1," "Restroom," "Lounge")
- Comment cards
- Invitations for grand opening

You can create some of the printed items yourself and have them printed at your local office supply store or local printer. Those items include the following:

- Patient chart sheets, such as progress notes, patient data sheet, exam sheets, and medication records
- Patient information sheets, such as instructions, diagnosis information, and medication information
- Super bill—charge sheet for the patient's visit (includes diagnosis and procedural codes)

Prescription pads can be ordered from a medical printing supply company or ordered free of charge from *Triple I Prescription Pads* in Cherry Hill, New Jersey, Tel: 1-800-969-7237).

Laboratory Fees   Check with three different laboratories for fees on the most common test you will be performing. Many laboratories will provide you with free supplies. Find out what they will provide and what they won't. Some will even provide you with a printer in your office so that you can get your lab reports faster.

Payroll   Ugh! How much are you planning to pay your employees? Don't count on a paycheck for yourself for a year or two. If you can afford to pay yourself sooner, great, but don't plan on it.

Payroll Taxes   Your accountant can teach you how to figure this amount. If you can estimate how much you will be paying your employees, then your accountant can tell you how much and how often you will need to pay payroll tax.

Sales Tax   If you are selling products, you may need to collect and pay state sales tax. Every state is different.

Professional Fees   Call your attorney for an estimate for incorporating your business. You will have accounting fees for setting up your books and helping you set up your tax schedules.

Health Insurance   Everyone's situation is different. If you are going to need to purchase health insurance, check around and evaluate the different policies. For now, you can estimate how much per month you will need to pay. Will you have to provide insurance for your employees? These costs add up fast, and you may need to negotiate the insurance costs with your employees for the first few years.

Liability Insurance   Many states require liability insurance for nurse practitioners. Know how much you are paying each year.

Disability Insurance   Depending on your situation, you may want to consider disability insurance. If you have family members that depend on your income to live, you may want to investigate this costly insurance.

Continuing Education   You can probably estimate this cost by looking at your continuing education costs over the past few years. It is important to keep current, but it is also very important to keep the costs in order. Your first year or two in business, you may want to bypass out-of-town conferences and earn your continuing education hours locally.

Entertainment and Promotions   This may be difficult to estimate, but put some numbers down. Plan on at least one lunch and one dinner a month to help you network and grow your business. You may want to figure in costs for holiday cards, promotional items, thank you cards, and the like.

Auto   Speak with your accountant regarding your transportation. Your accountant can help you decide how to handle this aspect of your business. Once your business is up and running, you may have your practice buy or lease your transportation. The business may also be able to cover the cost of fuel, insurance, and maintenance expenses as well.

Association Dues   Total up all of your association and organization dues. You may be surprised how much you are spending for dues. Belonging to associations and supporting growth for your profession are very important and many have super benefits.

Subscriptions   You will need to have current magazines in your waiting area. You should also keep current with good journals. Write in what you currently spend on journals and then what you think you will spend on waiting room magazines.

The total of your estimate of initial costs will give you an idea of how much money you may need to access to launch your practice. Once you have estimated your monthly costs, you can set goals for monthly (even weekly) income.

This may all seem a bit overwhelming, but you must have an idea of what the real costs of running a practice are before you make the commitment to start your practice.

ESTIMATING YOUR INCOME

This may be a difficult, but important, exercise. Only you know how many patients you can see in a day. Your specialty and location will have an effect on how much you can charge for your services. At this point, you should "guesstimate" (a combination of guessing and estimating!) how much in fees you will be able to bring in during your first months and year.

You may be planning to keep a per-diem position with an employer to help with the start-up cost during the first few months. You can include that in your projected income. Take a look at Figure 3–2 and start "guesstimating!"

Pencil in how much you think you will be charging for a regular visit and how many regular visits you can do in an 8-hour day, then multiply the two and the product is an estimate of how much money you can bring in during 1 day. Although, this may seem a bit unrealistic during the early stages of your practice, you can use this formula to determine whether you will be able to cover the overhead costs of your practice once you get going. Then, using the same formula, you can estimate how much you could bring in during 1 week and 1 month.

List all special procedures, laboratory tests, injections, and immunizations that your practice will be offering. Estimate how many special procedures you can do during the different time frames. You can combine the two: for example, five regular exams plus two Depo-Provera shots, five wet smears, 1 urinalysis, and so on. Think about what you are doing during a day's time in your current practice setting. Make this exercise as realistic as possible. Special procedures can enhance your revenues significantly. Most practices figure laboratory charges as three to four times what the laboratory charges to run the tests. That helps cover the staff and collection expenses. If your practice will offer injections and immunizations, survey the community for what is being charged locally.

Will you have any other income? Per-diem or part-time employment, teaching, renting out extra office space, public speaking, research income? This extra income can really be helpful during the first few years.

WEIGHING IT ALL OUT

Keeping in mind that the figures you have produced are estimates, you may now calculate your projected income or loss for certain periods of time. You will also have to determine how you will pay for your "initial costs."

Figure 3-2   **Estimated Income Worksheet.**

Basic Formula:

$_____ per visit   × _____ visits per day   = $_____ 1 day's income

#_____ visits per week   × $_____ per visit   = $_____ weekly income

#_____ visits per month   × $_____ per visit   = $_____ est. monthly income

Other Factors to Add in:

Special procedures

Laboratory income

Injections

Other income

Projected Monthly Income

- Visits $_____
- Special procedures $_____
- Laboratory income $_____
- Injections $_____
- Other Income $_____

Total income: $_____

Projected 6-Month Income

	January	February	March	April	May	June
Visits	$____	$____	$____	$____	$____	$____
Special Procedures	$____	$____	$____	$____	$____	$____
Laboratory Income	$____	$____	$____	$____	$____	$____
Injections	$____	$____	$____	$____	$____	$____
Other Income	$____	$____	$____	$____	$____	$____
Total Income:	$____	$____	$____	$____	$____	$____

Your estimated monthly costs can be compared with your estimated monthly income. You can play with these figures and find the minimum number of visits needed to cover the overhead costs for your office. You will want to know how much income you need for 1 week and 1 month. Then you can keep close tabs on things just by looking at your weekly bank deposit.

With these figures, you can project your income/loss for your first 6 or 12 months. This information is necessary for writing your business plan.

FINANCING YOUR VENTURE

On Figure 3–1 you calculated your estimated *initial costs*. This is the minimum amount you will need to secure before you can open your doors. Depending on your situation, you may want to add on several months of overhead costs or just a cushion of extra money to carry you over. There are many different ways to access this money and there are many different theories on which is the best way to access your start-up money. Sometimes, the easiest is not the smartest. For example, opting to use your credit card rather than applying for a loan may cost you more. The percentage rate of interest for your credit card will probably be twice what a loan would cost.

Think about your connections. Do you have family members who would extend a loan for your start-up money? Do you have it in your savings account? Do you have a house or other property you could use as collateral? Do you know someone who may want to invest in your practice for a percentage of ownership? There are many different lending centers and they all have their own applications and requirements. Many of the lending institutions are interested in lending money to new entrepreneurs. It may take a lot of investigating and repetitive work, but financing can be found. Most lenders are going to ask you for your *business plan*.

PREPARING A BUSINESS PLAN

Many people skip this vital step when designing their new business. The business plan is the working "care plan" of the development of your practice. Using this tool, you will think through many aspects of your business that you may not have thought about before. There are many books and computer programs available to help you write your business plan. There are even professionals who can help you, although this is going to be your business and it is best if you write the business plan yourself. How can the professional writer know everything about your dream practice? If you are going to use the business plan to acquire funding, a professional may be used to fine-tune your plan and give it a more professional appearance. The length and depth of this plan is up to you. The more information the better, but don't let it slow you down. Ready to get started?

To effectively analyze the potential of your proposed venture, you will have to make key decisions in order to define and illustrate the nature of your business. Now is the time to project and assess the financial viability of establishing an independent practice. Preparing a business plan will not only help you manage your new venture, but it is often used to raise money to finance your company. Therefore, it is best to develop a business plan before you hang that "open for business" sign outside your office.

There is an endless supply of excellent books and computer software that will help you prepare a formal business plan, and they all specify the following elements as integral parts of the document:

- *Statement of Purpose, Summary Statement, or Mission Statement,* which is an overview or concise description of your proposed practice.
- *Company Organization,* which specifies the type or form of company and how it will be managed and staffed. Give a brief description of the office and equipment.
- *Market Analysis,* which provides information on the services that you plan on providing, market size, clients, competition, and trends.
- *Financial Data,* which includes projections and estimates of expenses, income, and cash flow. Describe accounting systems and controls. Include the total finance required to fund the business.
- *Marketing Strategy,* which outlines your marketing philosophy, plans and methods. Include what distinguishes you from the competition.
- *Supporting Documents or Appendices,* which provide evidence to back up what you have stated in your proposal. Include financial forecasts (e.g., projected cash flow, profit and loss, balance sheets). Include any other relevant documents that demonstrate that you will have a successful business.

The length or depth of the plan really depends on where you will be using the plan. If it is just for your own planning, it may look a bit different than if you are presenting it to venture capitalists for financing. Preparing a business plan is to many the most important step in formulating or shaping a business idea into reality. This document helps you make key decisions regarding the nature and structure of your practice, as well as guiding you in managing your business. Investigate computer programs or books on writing your business plan so that you find one that is easy for you to use. Many have more detail than is really necessary. Use the Internet to gather information on different software and books.

THE FORM OR STRUCTURE OF YOUR BUSINESS

From the business end, you will need to decide the "form" or "structure" of your business. This is basically the legal form your new business will take.

There are three basic types or forms a new business can take, each with its own advantages and disadvantages. Even though this is a major decision, it is a decision that can be changed later on. Many firms start as one type or form and over time evolve into another. Numerous books and articles have been written on the different forms of business. In investigating this area, please note that there are tax and legal implications to all different forms of business—and there may be differences at the state level. Once your attorney or accountant has a full understanding of your proposed practice, he or she can guide you into the correct structure of your business.

The three basic forms of business are:

1. Sole proprietorship. This is an unincorporated business that is owned by one individual. This form is the most common for new businesses. Although it may be easy to establish and operate a business as a sole proprietor, there are financial risks to this approach, which should be considered. In essence, the assets of the individual owner could be in jeopardy if the business runs into trouble.

2. Partnership. A partnership is the relationship between two or more persons who join to carry on a trade or business. This form offers more financial security than the sole proprietorship. A partnership has more than one owner and all partners are liable for the acts of all the partners—provided that they were acting on behalf of the partnership. It is usually recommended that a partnership agreement be established early on to define the relationship and responsibilities of the partners.

3. Corporation. Forming a corporation offers more legal protection than the sole proprietorship or partnership forms of business. Corporations are considered to be separate entities from the individuals who own and/or operate the business. On the downside, there are more overhead costs to this form of business. State laws differ in this area and everyone's situation is different, so you will need to consult with your accountant to help you decide which is most appropriate for you. There are different types of corporations, and your professional support will help decide which is right for you.

Once you have consulted with your accountant and decided what form your business will take, you will need to confer with your attorney to help you get your legal papers in order for your practice.

MARKET ANALYSIS

A market analysis is, basically, checking out your area to determine whether your services are needed. You can do this yourself or you can hire someone. You need to have the confidence that the practice you are designing will have

enough patients in the area to support it. The three basic rules that would justify opening a practice in an area that already has services provided by others
are:

1. The market is growing and will support additional companies, or
2. The market is not growing, rather it is not being adequately served by
   existing companies, or
3. You have uniqueness to offer—in other words, your proposed practice
   will be special and better than others in the community.

You need to have the confidence that there are enough patients with the
ability to pay in your community. Some of the questions you should think
about regarding the market include:

1. Who are my potential patients?
2. Where are they located?
3. Will location, price, service, quality, or even the personality of the practitioner and staff influence the patients?
4. How does the size of the total market (potential patients in your community) affect my potential business?
5. How will the patients pay for services? Is most of the area covered by
   one or two HMO/Insurance companies? Will they accept a nurse practitioner as a provider?

To have the complete picture of your area, you must also investigate the
competition. In assessing the competition, you could delve a little deeper than
just checking the Yellow Pages. What services do they provide? What are some
of the strengths and weakness of your competition? Think about how you can
gain an edge over your competition in meeting the needs of your potential
patients.

Additionally, you should evaluate any changes or trends in the marketplace. For example, is there an increase or decrease in demand for certain services or procedures? In short, the emerging entrepreneur should investigate not
only the current conditions of the market, but also social, economic, and
demographic indicators or trends in determining the potential of a business.

LEGAL AND FINANCIAL CONSIDERATIONS

Legal and financial record keeping is a very important task for the entrepreneur. You need to create an effective filing and storage system. You need to be
able to locate your important papers easily when you need them. Regulations
differ from state to state, but some of the important legal and financial papers
you may need to keep track of include:

- Lease or property purchase agreements
- Incorporation papers
- Tax identification numbers
- Insurance policy information and cover sheets
- City, county, state, and federal licenses
- Signed contracts
- Protocol or supervision agreement
- Nurse practitioner license
- Collaborating or supervising physician license
- Patient records
- Biohazard waste permit
- Previous years' tax returns
- Continuing education documentation
- CLIA (Clinical Laboratory Improvement Act) certificate
- Occupational Safety and Health Administration documents
- Medicare and Medicaid provider numbers

You will also need to locate a good corporate attorney to help you establish your practice and maintain your legal records. A good certified public accountant is also a good find. Over the years, their expertise can be invaluable.

Now that you have collected and analyzed data regarding your projected income and expenses, you can make some major decisions—continue on or scrap the project. Remember, you can find your way around any obstacle if you try hard enough. An analysis of the potential of your business will help you highlight potential risks and contribute to the eventual success of your practice. Drawing up a thorough business description, analyzing the market, and carefully calculating the financial data will demonstrate that your new company is a well thought out venture. The business plan can prove not only to you but also to others that your practice will be successful.

SUGGESTIONS AND TIPS FROM WOMEN'S HEALTH WATCH, INC.

- Before you hire an attorney or accountant, do your homework. Some are better than others in dealing with small businesses and medical practices. Ask around; you may be able to get some great leads from other practitioners in your area. When you do call a meeting with a professional, it is in your best interest to be organized. Know exactly what you are going to ask and have a written agenda. Remember, these professionals charge by the minute, so make the most of your time—and get your money's worth!

▪ Tempting as it may be, do not bypass writing a business plan—even if it is just in your notebook for your eyes only. You really need to know what your monthly expenses will be and whether you will be able to cover them.

PERSONAL ANECDOTES

1. When trying to define my "target market," I decided that it would be "women ages 15 to 65." After doing a chart review of my first year, I found that my youngest patient was 7 years old; my oldest was 88! I even had male patients. So, I guess my original thoughts on my "target market" were a bit off.

2. When I was designing my practice, I asked a good friend if she would work as my "office manager." She agreed and I was pleased. I then started to get nervous. I felt like I needed to have the confidence that I could pay her on a regular basis. She was leaving a good job to come work for me. I figured out that if I continued working for my collaborating physician for 2 half days a week at a per-diem rate, I would make what I had agreed to pay her for a week. It made me feel a lot better knowing that I would not hurt a friend by not being able to pay her.

Resources

Covello, J,.and Hazelgren, BJ: The Complete Book of Business Plans: Simple Steps to Writing a Powerful Business Plan. Financial Sourcebooks, New York, 1994.

O'Donnell, M: Writing Business Plans that Get Results: A Step by Step Guide. NTC/Contemporary Publishing, Lincolnwood, IL, 1999.

Tiffany, P, and Peterson, SD: Business Plans for Dummies. IDG Books Worldwide, Foster City, CA, 1997.

Software

Business Plan Pro 4.0, Palo Alto Software.
Business Plan Toolkit (Mac), Palo Alto Software.
Smart Business Plan 8.0, Smart Online, Inc.

NOTES

Designing Your Practice

Chapter 4

Business Strategies and Development: How Do I Start a Practice?

" The method of the enterprising is to plan with audacity and execute with vigor "

Christian Bovée

Now that you have analyzed the potential of your business, it is time to start filling in the missing pieces. Good planning is critical for success in business. Knowing where you want to go with your business and how you intend to get there will ultimately contribute to your receiving a return on your investment. The more obvious decisions are no more or less important than the more difficult decisions. You are creating an entire package for success. Try to think through everything related to your practice down to the smallest detail.

BUSINESS EDUCATION

Ideally, one would complete the course work for a master's of business administration degree before launching into independent practice. However, that may not be realistic. Most nursing school curriculums do not include business courses. Of course, the more business education and experience, the better. If you do not have business education or experience, that does not mean you cannot run a successful practice. You just need to be aware that you may need to rely on professional assistance while you learn the ropes.

There are many ways to learn about business. Your local community college or university may have courses for individuals contemplating entrepreneurship. Some have *Small Business Institutes* that are organized through the Small Business Administration (SBA). The institutes provide counseling by students and faculty to small business clients. The institutes are located on more than 500 college campuses nationwide. A crash course on basic bookkeeping at a local college or even a more general course on business management would be beneficial.

The federal government created the *United States Small Business Administration* in 1953. The mission of the SBA is "to aid, council, assist, and protect the interests of small business concerns, to preserve free competitive enterprise, and to maintain and strengthen the overall economy of our nations." Your local SBA office has many workshops, programs, literature, and other resources designed to help the new entrepreneur establish and operate a new business. The SBA has a great Website, *www.sba.gov*, which contains helpful business information. The Service Corps of Retired Executives (SCORE) provides free counseling through the SBA. The SBA also helps with business financing. You can view and print the loan forms from the Website. The SBA has an extensive selection of information on many business management topics, from how to start a business to exporting your products. This information is listed in *The Small Business Directory.* The directory is free and available at your local SBA office. See Table 4–1 to locate your SBA State District Offices. It is definitely worth a call to see what they have to offer.

Another way to learn is to read. Business journals and magazines are excellent resources. You may not want to read them cover-to-cover, but scan the table of contents for articles that may be relevant to your business. Your local newspaper is a good resource. It is good to know what is going on in your community. The business section of the paper may have a calendar of events with business group meetings and events. The business associations usually have educational speakers and programs at their meetings.

There are many books, textbooks, and manuals on all aspects of small business available. You can find them at your library or online. Just like many parts of our educational process, this is up to you to investigate independently.

American Express has created a division called the *American Express Small Business Service.* They have created an online community that has small business news, online chats, and a broad range of small business resources. This Website can be found at *www.americanexpress.com/voices*.

What you have learned from your experiences with other practices or businesses concepts will help you run your own practice. There are many different ways to handle the business of your practice. Be open for change, and try different approaches. Just because you saw something done one way at a practice does not necessarily mean that is the best or only way. Design your practice the way you think it should be designed. Do not be tempted to take shortcuts that are not legal—you will regret it.

Whether you learn the ins and outs of business through formal educational courses or on the job, the important thing is to pay attention. Learn from the experiences of others as well as from your own experience. This is an area in which you should never stop learning and growing.

Table 4-1	The U.S. Small Business Administration (SBA)

Alabama
2121 8th Ave. North
Birmingham, AL 35203-2398
205-731-1344

Arizona
2828 N. Central Ave.
Phoenix, AZ 85004-1093
602-745-7200

California
660 J St., Suite 215
Sacramento, CA 95814-2499
916-498-6410

Connecticut
330 Main St., 2nd Floor
Hartford, CT 06106-1800
860-240-4700

Delaware
824 N. Market St.
Wilmington, DE 19801-3011
302-573-6294

Georgia
233 Peachtree St., NE, Suite 1900
Atlanta, GA 30303
404-331-0100

Idaho
1020 Main St.
Boise, ID 83702
208-334-1696

Indiana
429 N. Pennsylvania St., Suite 100
Indianapolis, IN 46204-1873
317-226-7272

Kansas
271 W. Third St., North, Suite 2500
Wichita, KS 67202-1212
316-269-6616

Louisiana
365 Canal St., Suite 2250
New Orleans, LA 70130-1112
504-589-2705

Maryland
10 South Howard St.
Baltimore, MD 21201
410-962-4392

Michigan
477 Michigan Ave., Suite 515
Detroit, MI 48226
313-226-6075

Mississippi
210 E. Capitol St., Suite 900
Jackson, MS 39201
601-965-4378

Montana
301 South Park, Room 334, Dr. 10054
Helena, MT 59626
406-441-1081

Nevada
300 Las Vegas Blvd. S., Suite 1100
Las Vegas, NV 89101
702-388-6611

Alaska
222 West 8th Ave.
Anchorage, AK 99513-7559
907-271-4022

Arkansas
2120 Riverfront Drive, Suite 100
Little Rock, AR 72202-1794
501-324-5871

Colorado
721 19th St., Suite 400
Denver, CO 80202
303-844-2607

District of Columbia
1110 Vermont Ave. NW, 9th Floor
Washington, DC 20005
202-606-4000

Florida
7825 Baymeadows Way, Suite 100B
Jacksonville, FL 32256
904-443-1900

Hawaii
300 Ala Moana Blvd., Room 2-235
Honolulu, HI 96850
808-541-2990

Illinois
500 W. Madison St., Suite 1250
Chicago, IL 60661-2511
312-353-4528

Iowa
210 Walnut St., Room 749
Des Moines, IA 50309
515-284-4422

Kentucky
600 Dr. MLK Jr. Place
Louisville, KY 40202
502-582-5761

Maine
40 Western Ave.
Augusta, ME 04330
207-622-8274

Massachusetts
10 Causeway St., Room 265
Boston, MA 02222-1093
617-478-4133

Minnesota
100 N. 6th St.
Minneapolis, MN 55403-1563
612-370-2324

Missouri
815 Olive St., Room 242
St. Louis, MO 63101
314-539-6600

Nebraska
11141 Mill Valley Road
Omaha, NE 68154
402-221-3606

New Hampshire
143 North Maine St., Suite 202
Concord, NH 03301
603-225-1400

[Continued]

Table 4–1	**The U.S. Small Business Administration (SBA)** *[Continued]*

New Jersey
Two Gateway Center, 15th Floor
Newark, NJ 07102
973-645-2434

New York
26 Federal Plaza, Suite 3100
New York, NY 10278
212-264-4354

North Dakota
657 Second Ave., N., Room 2192
Fargo, ND 58108
701-239-5131

Oklahoma
210 Park Ave., Suite 1300
Oklahoma City, OK 73102
405-231-5521

Pennsylvania
900 Market St., 5th Floor
Philadelphia, PA 19107-4228
215-580-2SBA

South Carolina
1835 Assembly St., Room 358
Columbia, SC 29201
803-765-5377

Tennessee
50 Vantage Way, Suite 201
Nashville, TN 37228
615-736-5881

Utah
125 South State St., Room 2231
Salt Lake City, UT 84138
801-524-3209

Virginia
400 North 8th St., Suite 1150
Richmond, VA 23240
804-771-2400

West Virginia
320 West Pike St., Suite 330
Clarksburg, WV 26301
304-623-5631

Wyoming
100 East B St., Room 4001
Casper, WY 82602
307-261-6500

New Mexico
625 Silver, SW, Suite 320
Albuquerque, NM 87102
505-346-7909

North Carolina
200 N. College St., Suite A2015
Charlotte, NC 28202
704-344-6563

Ohio
Nationwide Plaza, Suite 1400
Columbus, OH 43215
614-469-6860

Oregon
1515 SW Fifth Ave., Suite 1050
Portland, OR 97201-5494
503-326-2682

Rhode Island
380 Westminster St.
Providence, RI 02903
401-528-4561

South Dakota
110 S. Phillips Ave., Suite 200
Sioux Falls, SD 57104-6727
605-330-4231

Texas
4300 Amon Carter Blvd., Suite 114
Fort Worth, TX 75155
817-684-5500

Vermont
87 State St., Room 205
Montpelier, VT 05601
802-828-4422

Washington
801 W. Riverside, Suite 240
Spokane, WA 99201
509-353-2800

Wisconsin
740 Regent St., Suite 100
Madison, WI 53715
608-441-5263

PROFESSIONAL SUPPORT

When initiating the search for professional support, ask your colleagues for referrals. It will save a lot of time, energy, and money if you can identify professionals who have a good understanding of the nurse practitioner's role. If you do not find a professional who knows about nurse practitioners, you will spend time and money educating him or her on the role of the nurse practitioner. You may also not get the correct guidance if they don't truly understand what you are going to be doing. If you cannot locate professionals who have worked with nurse practitioners, look for someone who has worked with medical practices. That is better than working with someone who has no medical professional clients.

Corporate Attorney It is comforting to engage an attorney who knows you and understands your practice. Your attorney will be able to assist you in making decisions regarding your corporation and personal business. Your attorney guides you if legal concerns arise. Unexpected roadblocks could possibly escalate into major problems if not handled appropriately in a timely fashion. You may want to use your attorney for more personal things, such as preparing your will and helping with real estate transactions. Hopefully, you will never have to contact a "malpractice attorney," but you should be prepared just in case you are sued. Learn who the successful medical malpractice attorneys are in your area. Narrow down the list to the attorneys who represent physicians and other medical professionals. Even better is to find an attorney who is also a nurse practitioner. (Yes, there are some out there!) Keep this name and number handy, although the choice of attorney may be out of your hands depending on the stipulations of your liability insurance. Your first call, if you are being sued, is to your insurance carrier, who will guide you through this horrific process.

Certified Public Accountant (CPA) Your relationship with your CPA can be invaluable, even before you start your practice. Your CPA can help you get your accounting software set up properly with your chart of accounts. Your CPA may have some ideas and leads for you in locating start-up financing. You can work together in setting financial goals. You will want to set up a calendar with tax due dates. The last thing you want to do is to get in trouble with the Internal Revenue Service. Your CPA can teach you not only how to generate reports through your accounting software but also how to interpret the reports. There are certain papers you will need to prepare and compile at the end of the year for your tax return preparation. Your CPA can guide you through this process.

Marketing Consultant Whether you feel the need to launch a true marketing blitz or you just need help mapping out a plan, a marketing consultant will be able to help you. The expertise of a marketing consultant may help you get the word out on your new practice faster and in a more cost-effective manner than if you try it on your own. This may be money well spent or possibly money wasted. Interview any prospective marketing consultants and weigh the costs versus the benefits of working with them.

CHOOSING A BUSINESS NAME AND LOGO

Choosing the name of your practice can be fun, or it can be painful. You may feel rushed to decide on a name because you must have a name before you can incorporate your business. Your main goal is to develop a name for your practice that will be easily remembered and recognized. You want your patients to be able to find you easily if they misplace your card. Designing a logo can help them recognize your practice as well.

To create the name of your practice, start by writing down a few things. First, who will your patients be? Children, adults, women, men, the elderly? You may want to use the name of your target market in your practice name. You will also want to define how you want your practice recognized. What does the word "clinic" mean to you? Is that a good descriptor for your practice? How about "health center?" Look through the Yellow Pages. See if there are any words that you definitely do want to include in the name. Or, are there any words you do not want in the name? If you have a simple last name, you may want to incorporate it into the name of your practice. However, if your last name is long or difficult to say or spell, you might do better using another name. You want to make it easy for the patient to locate you. Start listing out potential names, then test them on family members, friends, and colleagues. One name should stick out and make you feel good. Is it a good descriptor of your intended practice? If you have trouble with this exercise, ask your friends and family to help you. This is a decision that will be with you as long as you have your practice. Don't make the name too specific in case your practice grows in another area. (At Women's Health Watch, we started to see male patients—they may have felt a little funny walking into Women's Health Watch!) Your attorney may ask you to submit possibly three potential names for your practice. A search will be done to find the name that is not already in use in your state. Be sure to write the names in the order of preference. Once you have decided on the three potential names of your practice, you can schedule with your attorney to get your business papers in order (incorporation).

Developing a logo for your practice is not a necessity, but it is yet another way to help your patients recognize your practice. Your logo can be included on your business cards, letterhead, signs, all advertising, and in the Yellow Pages. Over the years, people may recognize you from the logo—just think of the big yellow arches you see in front of a restaurant or the peacock on television.

PROTOCOLS AND LICENSURE

To operate an independent practice as a nurse practitioner, you *must* know the laws in your state. Many states require written management protocols be created, signed (by the nurse practitioner and collaborating physician), and submitted to the Board of Nursing. Every state is different. A few states do not require physician collaboration. You must do your research and follow the laws explicitly.

If your state requires that a written protocol be developed, check with your governing board for the suggested format. There are different theories regarding how specific you should be in defining your practice within your protocol.

Some think you should outline exactly what patients you will be seeing, what procedures you will be performing, what drugs you will be prescribing, and so on. Some nurse practitioners have gone so far as to name a textbook and state that they will follow the practices outlined in the book. That could be too limiting. Think about what could happen if the book recommended one treatment for an ailment and you prescribed another. Even if the treatment you prescribed was safe and well known, your action would still be in violation of your protocol. A more broad description seems more forgiving.

Experts say protocols can be used against nurse practitioners in the case of a malpractice suit, so be very careful with your wording. Remember to update your protocol when you master a new skill or start prescribing a new classification of medication. Many states require that the protocol be updated on a yearly basis. Put it on your calendar. You do not want to be found delinquent in any area. A sample of a protocol is shown in Table 4–2.

Some states also require notification be sent to the Board of Medicine on a yearly basis outlining your collaborative relationship with your collaborating physician. Learn what your state requirements are and follow the law to the letter (Box 4–1).

The state licensure requirements vary from state to state as well. Whatever your state requirements are for initial licensing and renewal are very important to learn. Keep on your calendar your renewal dates and the continuing education requirements (if needed) so that you can keep current. Some states require special educational courses for renewal in areas such as domestic violence, HIV updates, and child abuse. It is up to you to keep track of what is required and when it is due. Devise a system that works for you. One of the worst feelings one can experience is to receive a notice of a license audit when you have not done what you were supposed to do.

Box 4–1

December 5, 1999

Board of Medicine
Department of Professional Regulation
1940 North Monroe St., Suite 60
Tallahassee, FL 32399-0750

To Whom It May Concern:

Please be advised that (*physician's name*) and (*nurse practitioner's* name) are working in collaboration in the specific management areas as stated in her protocol of practice.

Nurse practitioner's name	Date	FL License Number
Physician's name	Date	FL License Number

Table 4-2	**Advanced Registered Nurse Practitioner Management Protocol**

NAME: Your Name, Degrees

ADDRESS: Street Address

City, State, Zip Code

LICENSE: XXXXXXX

Protocol effective date: January 1, 2001

EMPLOYED BY: (Multiple employers, please see location sites)

ARNP SIGNATURE: _____

MEDICAL DOCTOR: _____

Physician's Name, MD

FL License #XXXXXXX

I.   Requiring Authority:

Nurse Practice Act, Florida Statute, Chapter 464 Florida Board of Nursing Rules Chapter 210–11 and 210–16, Administrative Policies Pertaining to Advanced Registered Nurse Practitioners, Florida Administrative Code.

II.   General Identifying Data:

A.   Individuals part to protocol

1.   Name of Individual, Degrees

Certified as an Advanced Registered Nurse Practitioner, Certificate Number XXXXXXX, as issued by the Florida Board of Nursing (see attached).

2.   Physician's Name, MD, Florida License Number XXXXXXX, DEA Number XXXXXXXXX.

B.   Specialty: Adult Health, including obstetrics and gynecology (women's health)

C.   Sites: Women's Health Watch, Inc.

4540 North Federal Hwy.

Fort Lauderdale, FL 33308

Women's Clinic

2331 North State Road 7, Suite 104

Fort Lauderdale, FL 33313

D.   Date of Protocol Development: December 05, 2000

III.   Scope of Practice: In collaboration with *Physician's Name,Individual's Name* will assess and manage the general health status for those clients for which she has been educated and trained, specifically in adult health, including obstetrics and gynecology (women's health).

IV.   Specific Management Areas:

A.   The following measures may be initiated and/or conducted by *Individual's Name*

1.   Comprehensive history and physical assessments, with emphasis on thyroid, heart, lung, abdomen, pelvic exam (including Pap smear, cultures, and other laboratory tests as indicated).

2.   The following procedures under the indirect supervision and delegation by *Physician's Name*

a.   Insert and remove intrauterine devices

b.   Insert, fit, and remove diaphragms

c.   Insert, fit, and remove pessaries

d.   Insert Dilapan or Laminaria (cervical dilation treatment) as directed by Physician

e.   Insert and remove Norplant contraceptive systems

f.   Excise mucosal and skin lesions

g.   Treat condylomata with BCA or TCA

h.   Order radiographic studies as indicated

i.   Provide HIV pre- and post-test counseling

j.   Order any laboratory work or patient care as indicated

k.   Perform ultrasound pregnancies for gestational measurement

l.   Perform colposcopy with cervical and endocervical biopsies

m.   Perform cryosurgery of the cervix

n.   Conduct endometrial biopsies

Table 4-2	**Advanced Registered Nurse Practitioner Management Protocol** *[Continued]*

o. Perform sclerotherapy of varicosities and telangiectasias

p. Conduct any other procedure for which the ARNP has been educated and trained.

3. Development and prescribing of diagnostic and therapeutic plans with the supervision and/or consultation of *Physician's Name*.

4. Consultations with physicians and health professionals.

B. The following drug therapies may be prescribed, monitored, initiated or altered by *Individual's Name*, in accordance with education and management protocols: anti-inflammatory agents, antiarthritics, analgesics, antibiotics, antibacterials, antiparasitics, local anesthetics, vaccinations, antihistamines, antifungals, antitussives, antivirals, laxatives, diuretics, decongestants, bronchodilators, expectorants, contraceptives, dermatologicals, fertility agents, muscle relaxants, uterine relaxants, antacids, antianemics, antidiarrheals, antiemetics, antithyroid agents, antiulcer agents, lipid lowering agents, hormones, antihypertensives, oral hypoglycemics, smoking cessation medicines, vitamins, herbs, and minerals.

C. Other responsibilities the ARNP may perform under the direct and indirect supervision of the physician include:

1. Case management of clients in office

2. Health education to clients and their families

3. Continuing education in specialty area

4. Communication with physician for review and evaluation of professional performance

5. Maintenance of current licensure as ARNP by the State of Florida Board of Nursing

6. Access to the supervising physician or substitute at all times.

V. Supervision:

A. This protocol shall be reviewed on an annual basis and amended as required.

B. All of the above functions may be performed under general supervision.

C. A copy of the protocol and a copy of the notice required by the Board of Medicine will be kept at the site of practice. After the termination of the relationship between *Individual's Name* and *Physician's Name*, each party will be responsible for ensuring that a copy of the protocol is maintained for future reference for 4 years as required.

X

_____

Individual's Name, Degrees   Date   License #

X

_____

Physician's Name, MD   Date   License #

Appendices (to be kept within the ARNP practice site):

A. CVs or resumes of all parties.

B. Management protocols pertaining to care of clients.

C. Other resource materials used by the ARNP.

General:

A. The original of the protocol shall be filed with the Board of Nursing yearly. A copy will be stored at all practice sites.

B. Any alteration or amendments should be signed by all parties and filed with the Board of Nursing within 30 days of the alteration.

Address
Board of Nursing
4080 Woodstock Drive, Suite 202
Jacksonville, FL 32207

C. The notice required by the Board of Medicine 458.348(1) shall be filed yearly.

Address
Board of Medicine
Department of Professional Regulation
1940 North Monroe Street, Suite 60
Tallahassee, FL 32399-0750

DEVELOPING YOUR BUSINESS

Keeping all your notes and plans in order at this stage of development is critical. You need to be able to recall all the information you have gathered when you need it. You also need to keep current lists of "things to do." Keep lists of questions you need to ask certain people (accountant, lawyer, marketing consultant, collaborating physician, landlord). The organizational system you design for your planning notes should work for you (e.g., keep a binder with dividers or a portable filing system). Many of the things you are trying to accomplish depend on other things you have to get done first. You may feel that it is the "one step forward, three steps back" game. Hang in there and keep plodding along. Review your lists daily and accomplish as much as you can each day.

The actual development of your business is an ongoing process. You will not be done until you no longer own your practice. Keep asking yourself how you could be doing better, not only with patient care but also with improving your business and revenues.

SELECTING A PRACTICE LOCATION

If you have not decided on a city or state where you will start your practice, you may want to assess the saturation level of practitioners in the cities you are considering. The American Medical Association produces a reference book, *Physicians Characteristics and Distribution in the U. S.,* which may be helpful. This reference book may be available through your local library, hospital, or medical society. You could also assess how much growth can be expected by checking with the local hospital or city offices for the demographic data and projections for the area. If you are willing to relocate to an underserved area, check with the state and local health departments.

There are many differing theories on selecting your practice location. Ideally, you would work in a beautiful building with nice landscaping on a busy street. This ideal location would also include a huge lighted sign and a big parking lot. Being close to a mall and a high growth area would be nice. Having a bus stop, train stop, and a highway exit close by would be a plus. Having an office that is easy to find is important because your staff will be devoting quite a bit of time explaining to new patients how to get to your office. Then, reality sets in—what can you afford?

The safety of the neighborhood for your patients, staff, and yourself should be taken into consideration. Is there a security system installed? Do you feel you will need one?

How big of an office do you need to start with? You don't want to commit to a space that you may outgrow too quickly—what a wonderful problem that would be! How many exam rooms can you actually use? If there is just one of you, more than two exam rooms shouldn't be necessary. Is there enough room for your equipment and staff? Is designated parking available for you and your staff?

Compare rent charges from one space to another. Weigh it out. Which space will give you the best start? It may be better to pay a couple of hundred dollars more each month for a space that gives your practice more exposure.

LEASING VERSUS PURCHASING OFFICE SPACE

When considering a specific office space, you may find that you are able to purchase the office instead of just renting the space. You should investigate your options—you may have a nice surprise. If you have another property or collateral, purchasing the office may be a possibility. How much nicer in the long run it would be if you could be making a mortgage payment instead of a rent payment. Consult with your accountant about the benefits of personally purchasing the property and renting it to your practice. Many find this arrangement to be financially beneficial. You could be growing your personal assets while you are building your practice. One of the downsides of purchasing your office is that it may limit your future expansion and relocation.

If you are leasing, be sure to think through all of the details that you wish to have included in the lease—who will be responsible for what. Have your attorney give you guidance and review the lease before you sign it. Try to ask for more than you really expect to be included—for example, certain utilities, repairs, changes to the interior, landscaping, new flooring. You never know, the landlord may just go for it! Chances are the landlord will not volunteer to pay anything extra without your prompting. You may even offer to pay a little less than what is being asked. If the building has been vacant for a while, the landlord may accept your offer. Practice the art of negotiation. Make it fun. Try to keep your emotions out of this—think of it as a game.

SETTING UP YOUR OFFICE

First, walk through your office as if you were a patient coming in for a visit. Take notes so you know exactly what you need to buy and do. As clients walk in, is there an open area where the office staff can see them and greet them? Is there a place for them to sit while they fill out their information sheets? Are there clipboards and pens for the papers?

Then, walk back to where they will be going next. Is there a patient bathroom for sample collection? How are you going to handle those samples? Is there a pass-through window or will you have a tray where specimens can be placed? Now, where are they going to go? Into the laboratory area? Do you have a scale for obtaining height and weight? Do you have a chair where clients can sit during blood collection? Do you have a good workspace for papers and supplies, a blood pressure cuff, thermometer? Will they be going into the exam room next? Do you have the appropriate exam table, garbage cans, and supply cabinet? How about lighting? Do a mock exam—list the supplies you need to order.

Now that they are done with this hypothetical exam, the patient will need to "check out" at the front desk. What equipment will you need? Copy machine, credit card machine, calculator, computer, and typewriter? Are you going to give your patients your business card so they can find you again? Think about it. You want them not only to remember that you were very nice, caring, and competent, but also to call your office again.

The Internet has changed the way many Americans shop. You can use the Internet to find good deals on medical supplies as well as your office supplies and equipment. Compare prices. You may be able to save a lot of money shopping online (Box 4–2).

BUSINESS LICENSES

Learning what is required by your city, county, and state is your first step in getting organized with licenses. You can call the city, county, and state offices to learn the application process for the required business licenses. Your local SBA office will have this information available for you. You can save a lot of time and aggravation by consulting with the local SBA. Many of the licenses need to be renewed each year, so mark your calendar to stay current. The fire inspector may come around once a year to check the exit lights, emergency lighting, and fire extinguishers—be prepared. Biohazardous waste disposal may require a special license or certificate; this again may be state, county, or city regulated. It goes without saying that you will keep your nurse practitioner licensure up to date!

Box 4–2
Medical Supply Internet Sites

www.allegiancecorp.com	*www.medibuy.com*
www.empacthealth.com	*www.medicalbuyer.com*
www.equipmd.com	*www.medicalsuppliesusa.com*
www.esurg.com	*www.medline.com*
www.everythingformds.com	*www.medsite.com*
www.mdchoice.com	*www.neoforma.com*

All licenses should be posted in a space that is visible to your patients. If you are required to have a collaborative physician, then you should also post a copy of his or her medical license next to yours. A bulletin board is useful because you will be getting new licenses at renewal time.

If you are performing any type of laboratory testing (e.g., urine dip, urine pregnancy testing, wet smears), you must have a CLIA (Clinical Laboratory Improvement Act) certificate.

OVERVIEW OF REGISTRATIONS AND LICENSES

- Corporation papers—Whether you have created a corporation, partnership, or proprietorship, you must comply with state and federal laws governing the operation of your business. Initial filings, elections, and registrations are required by all practices, but the requirements vary with the type of entity you have started. This is an area for your attorney; he or she will know exactly what is required.

- Federal Identification Number—This number is required for all new businesses. You will be asked for this number by many different sources. To obtain your Federal Identification Number, you must file Form SS-4 with the Internal Revenue Service. Speak with your attorney; he or she may have done this for you when you started your corporation. If you need Form SS-4, it may be accessed through the Website *www.irs.ustreas.gov/prod/forms-pubs/*. Many states and municipalities also require a similar identification number.

- Your city and county may require you to register and obtain an occupational or business license from them. It is usually a simple procedure with a minimal fee. The licenses usually need to be renewed every 1 or 2 years. The fire marshall may have to inspect your office annually for adequacy of exit signs, emergency lighting, and fire extinguishers.

- Clinical Laboratory Improvement Act (CLIA) is a federal program that is administered by the Health Care Financing Administration (HCFA). This program was instituted, basically, to protect the citizens by regulating laboratory testing. A CLIA certificate is required for all laboratories, including small laboratories in health-care providers' offices. If you perform any testing (e.g., urine dips, finger sticks, microscopies), you must apply for a certificate. There are several levels of certificate based on the complexity of the testing you are performing. You may print the application for a CLIA certificate (Form HCFA–116) at *www.hcfa.gov/medicaid/clia/ cliaapp.htm*. For more information, write to the HCFA CLIA Program, P.O. Box 26689, Baltimore, MD 21207-0479. You must also contact your state agency to learn your state's requirements. You may locate information for your state agency at *www.hcfa.gov/medicaid/clia/ssa-map.htm.*

- Occupational Safety and Health Act (OSHA) was instituted to ensure safe and healthful working conditions for working men and women. All employers must comply with the OSHA standards for their business. These standards can be found at *www.osha.gov/.* You should also investigate what your state OSHA requirements entail. There are very specific rules regarding the handling of blood products, needles, glass capillary tubes, sharps disposal, biohazardous waste, and much more. There are requirements for labeling and handling chemicals in the office, employee training, and employee manuals. Independent businesses have been created that will train your employees, create a manual for your office, and help you comply with all of the rules. It may be worth the money to contract with one of these companies rather than put yourself at risk for hefty fines.

- You may be required to obtain a permit from the city, county, or state to operate as a Biohazardous Waste Generator—meaning you are producing biohazardous waste and disposing of it properly.

- Narcotics licenses are a requirement for the U. S. Department of Justice–Drug Enforcement Administration for those who administer, prescribe, or dispense drugs listed in the Controlled Substance Act. The legality of prescribing controlled substances by nurse practitioners varies from state to state. More information can be found at *www.deadiversion.usdoj.gov/drugreg/process.htm* or by calling 1-800-882-9539.

- Dispensing license may be required by your state if you are selling medications from your practice.

- Nurse practitioner license, protocol, national certification—don't forget the obvious! Keep on top of these; the last thing you need is trouble from something simple, such as not completing the required continuing education or not submitting appropriate forms and fees.

- CPR (cardiopulmonary resuscitation) certification or ACLS (advanced cardiac life support) training is a must for an independent practitioner. Don't let this lapse. Also, see that your employees stay current at least with basic first aid and CPR.

- Other. There may be other registrations and licenses required in your area. Check with other providers to make sure you have all of your bases covered.

Table 4–3 is a check-off sheet you can use to keep a record of your application status and renewal dates.

Table 4-3 Practice Regulations and License Check-Off Sheet

License Registration	Requested Application	Received Application	Submitted Application	License Received	Renewal Date
Corporation papers					
Federal I.D. Number					
City Occupational License					
County Occupational License					
Fire Marshall					
CLIA					
OSHA Handbook & Training					
Biohazard Waste					
Narcotics License					
Dispensing License					
Nurse Practitioner License					
Protocol Submitted					
National Certification					
CPR/ACLS for Self					
CPR and first aid for Employees					

RELATIONSHIPS

When dealing with representatives from laboratories, governmental agencies, and various inspectors, kindness is the key. Sometimes with the stresses of the day, it may be difficult to always put your best foot forward. However, with these people, building a friendship into your relationship will only benefit you. These people have the power. They make decisions that can affect your practice in many different ways. They can decide how much you will be paying for certain things, some can write citations with fines, and some even have the power to close down your practice. So, whenever a representative shows up, take a deep breath, put on a nice smile, and do your best to build a good friendship and business relationship.

PRACTICE REGULATIONS AND RELATIONSHIPS: WHAT ARE THE RULES?

When starting an independent practice, you will find there are more licenses and registrations required than you could have ever guessed. The rules are plenty, and you must be aware of them all. You must comply with all of the registrations, licenses, and regulations, or you may find yourself facing serious monetary fines, loss of licensure, and possibly, the closing of your practice.

The relationships you forge with laboratory representatives, inspectors, and representatives from governmental agencies can be critical for your success. Learning how to cultivate these relationships can make life a lot easier for you and your staff.

SMALL BUSINESS LOANS

If you completed the exercises in estimating your start-up costs in the preceding chapter, you should have an idea of how much money you will need to start your practice. You may also want to figure in extra to help cover expenses during the first 6 to 12 months. Hopefully, you won't need the extra money, but it is better to have access to capital than it is to run short.

There are many ways to locate the money needed to establish your practice. You may have the money available from your personal savings or credit line. If you own a house or property, you may be able to borrow against it. If you have already established a working relationship with a bank, then the bank may find a way to lend you the money. You may have friends or family who could lend you the money. When you are discussing your ideas for your practice with others, you may be able to identify a potential investor.

The local SBA office has information on loans. If you qualify for "minority status," more loans may be available to you. The definition of "minority" may differ between agencies, so you may want to investigate the definition.

You will need to know a few things about borrowing before you go to potential lenders. There are basically two types of loans: *lines of credit* and *installment loans*. There are two categories of loan length, *short-term* and *long-term*. A *line of credit* is an account with the bank similar to a personal credit card, but it is established for the business. There is a predetermined limit, and you can borrow up to that amount. You pay on the account similar to the credit card. You can pay off and borrow as often as you wish. Some lenders require that you bring the account balance down to zero once a year. Each bank will have different rules and fees. There is usually an annual fee and interest charged on what you owe.

An *installment loan* provides you with a certain lump sum and you pay it back on a regular payment schedule for a certain number of months, similar to making car payments.

Short-term loans are usually repaid within less than a year. It would be used for a certain project whose funding could be paid back quickly.

Long-term loans are usually paid back over a number of years. This type of loan is usually used for an improvement that will benefit the business and help increase revenues over time.

Here are some other terms used in the lending world that you should be aware of before you venture into talks with lenders. *Collateral* is usually something that you pledge to secure a loan. (In other words, if you fail to pay back the loan, they get to keep what you have pledged! So be careful.) Many types of collateral can be used to secure a loan. Sometimes just your signature and credit reputation are the only requirements needed to secure a loan. However, sometimes the bank requires a pledge of some or all of your assets to secure the loan. This is referred to as a *secured loan*. Some items used to secure loans include real estate, savings, equipment, stocks, and life insurance policies.

Venture capital firms are usually only interested in investment projects requiring an investment of $250,000 to 1,500,000. However, some may be more flexible. They are usually looking for a percentage (10% to 90%) of the business.

Some nonprofit organizations provide grants and loans to small business owners. One that has been discussed in the news media is *Count-Me-In.* This New York–based firm provides micro loans to women business owners (Box 4–3).

If you are planning to work with a lending institution, be prepared to fill out applications and financial reports. Because your business will not have a history or credit experience, the lender will most likely want to know everything about your personal finances for the past 2 years, including seeing your tax returns. The lender will also want a business plan that demonstrates how the business will be successful. This all may seem like a bothersome process, but it is probably the best way to access capital for your practice. You may learn more about your personal financial situation by completing the application process. You will probably have to complete a *Personal Financial Statement* that will give you your *personal net worth*. It is a great exercise to

Box 4–3
Start-Up Financing Grants and Loan Sources

www.americanexpress.com/voices—Small business information online community.

www.capitalsearch.net—Equity Net Angel Investor—private angel investors and venture capital sources ($50,000 and up).

www.countmein.com—Nonprofit organization that provides online micro (up to $5,000) loans to women business owners.

www.fastcash.com—Home equity, debt consolidation, home improvement loans, refinancing, home purchases. Bad credit O.K!

www.federal-government-grants.com—Grants to finance small business ventures.

www.fedmoney.com—Federal Money Retriever (grants and loans)—an interactive database covering all U.S. and government grant and loan programs. Includes a concise "Guide to Federal Funding."

www.firstunion.com/wbo—Online Women's Business Center. Loans available, 24 hour turn-around on loan decisions.

www.flashcommerce.com—Real-time small business loans. An e-commerce site looking for small business borrowers.

www.fleet.com/smallbusiness—Same day response to completed one page application.

www.hrsa.gov/bhpr/grants.html—Government grants for advance practice nurses working with schools of nursing, nursing centers, academic health centers, state or local governments, and other public or private nonprofit entities.

www.Inc.com—Research information on small business grants, insurance, and laws.

www.onlinewbc.org—Business information for women, micro lenders, and community banks that specialize in smaller loans with a focus on women and minority businesses. In-depth articles on all aspects of financing.

www.sba.gov—SBA loan information and assistance.

www.selfemploymentservice.com—The latest about government small business grants.

www.smallbusinessloans.com—2-Minute approval on small business loans or equipment leases. Money within 24 hours.

www.sweetsite.com—Finance center offers mortgage, home equity, credit card, automobile, and personal loans.

www.wellsfargo.com—Committed to lending $10 billion over 10 years to women owned business in the Western United States.

www.womeninc.com—A national nonprofit membership organization that provides financial services and member discounts on a variety of business services. Loans for women business owners.

complete annually even if it isn't required. It gives you good information—is your personal net worth increasing or declining?

There are many great Websites that contain invaluable financing information. LiveCapital corporate (*www.livecapital.com/getfinancing.html*) provides one-stop shopping for business loans, credit cards, and other financing from more than 70 major lenders around the country. With LiveCaptial you can apply for financing online for free. The Capitol Connection (*www. capitolconnection.com*) is a great resource for lending contacts and alternative financing.

APPEARANCE AND SAFETY OF THE OFFICE

First impressions... You know what they say! You want your patients to have the best possible first impression when they arrive at your office. It doesn't have to be decorated expensively by a designer; it just needs to be neat, clean, and comfortable. If your patients are going to have to sit and wait, let them be comfortable in a pleasant environment. Take a look around at some of the offices in town. It can be a real turn-off seeing stained or worn carpet and furniture in disrepair in the waiting room. Patients do assess the cleanliness of your office. They may not comment on it if they see cobwebs, dust, dirt, hair, or even medical waste on the floor. However, they may just decide never to come back.

When deciding on a color scheme for your office, think of warm, comforting colors. If you are seeing pediatric patients, you may opt for primary colors such as yellow or green. Many tones of blue and gray tend to give off a cold, depressive feeling. Think about what colors make you feel the most relaxed and comfortable—after all, you will be spending many hours in this space too!

Have a written daily and weekly cleaning schedule. Know who is responsible for which duties. Decide which chores need to be done at the end of each workday (e.g., all garbage cans emptied, coffee carafe washed, bathroom counters wiped down, lab surfaces washed). Then write out what should be done weekly (e.g., floors, sinks, dusting). If need be, make out check-off sheets for the cleaning duties and then have the assigned person check it off and return it to you or your office manager at a specified time. Then you will know who was responsible for the chore that wasn't done. When you first open your practice, you may want to have an employee assigned to do the cleaning. It is a great feeling when your patient says "Your office is always so clean!"

When walking through your office, think about any potential mishaps that could result from the environment. Ask yourself:

- Is the flooring intact?
- Are there handrails in the bathroom?

■ Are the parking lot, office, and patient bathroom wheelchair accessible?

Look for anything the patient could easily stumble over or get hurt by, and correct the situation before it becomes a problem. Even though you have given the office a thorough inspection, be prepared—accidents happen.

EMERGENCY PREPAREDNESS PLANNING

Think of some of the bad things that you know have happened to other businesses. Do your best to prevent a bad thing from turning into a horrible thing. Have your fire extinguishers in good repair and in a convenient location in case a fire starts. Have several telephones throughout the office so you can call 911 quickly. The exit signs and emergency lighting must be in good working order at all times. If the power goes out during a procedure, what will you do? Have flashlights ready!

What if a patient falls and loses consciousness? Do you have smelling salts handy? CPR mouth covers? Do you have a first-aid kit? Is your staff CPR trained? Talk with your staff about how you would like to handle certain situations—the last thing you need is extra panic from your staff.

SUGGESTIONS AND TIPS FROM WOMEN'S HEALTH WATCH, INC.

■ When negotiating employment with my future office manager, I offered to pay her a little extra to do the office cleaning. I explained what I expected and the cleaning schedule I preferred. She did a fantastic job of cleaning. She did a thorough cleaning on Mondays when I was not in the office and completed the daily cleaning I had requested. It worked out very well. You may want to consider an arrangement similar to this.

■ The expense of the creation of the Women's Health Watch logo was money well spent. I had the logo put on all printed materials and on the sign outside. People recognized it and commented on how distinctive it was. It also made the business look like a real business, that is, it adds to the professional appearance.

■ The National Association of Women Business Owners (NAWBO) in my community hosted monthly meetings with dynamic educational speakers on business. The contacts, referrals, and educational opportunities are endless with a group like NAWBO. You should research the business organizations in your area and attend some meetings. You can practice your networking skills while learning more about business.

■ Early on we developed a good friendship with the representatives from the laboratories we were using for our laboratory testing. When they got to know our patient base—and us—we were able to put together different screening programs at great prices. When we needed anything, there was a person we knew we could call upon. With a laboratory, that can be critical—sometimes we needed laboratory reports quickly, even when there were problems with billing or supplies. Because of the relationships we built, we were able to negotiate seriously low prices for all of our laboratory testing.

■ The office manager at Women's Health Watch, Inc., was responsible for keeping a special calendar of renewal dates. All of the licenses and registrations on Table 4–3 were kept on a calendar on her desk. We then had the confidence that we were on top of things and current with all of our licenses.

■ After about a year of struggling, trying to keep current on OSHA changes on our own, we learned of a company that was incredibly helpful. They knew everything there was to know about OSHA regulations for our practice. They inspected the office and made comments on things we needed to change or improve. They brought in the required educational materials and provided testing and certification. They compiled an appropriate OSHA office handbook. Once a year, they updated our records and our office handbook. Their fee was minimal compared to the time and aggravation we experienced trying to do this ourselves. Furthermore, if we were ever inspected by OSHA, they would be present to defend us. It gave us a lot of comfort knowing we had them in our court.

PERSONAL ANECDOTES

1. I did what all of the business experts advise you not to do. I financed the start-up of my practice with my VISA card. Ugh. Talk about high rates that go on and on. Take the time to investigate your potential to obtain a loan or a grant.

2. When trying to decide on a name for my future practice, I went so far as to check out-of-state telephone books for ideas. This confirmed my earlier thoughts that the name we had chosen was the best for my practice. For example, I didn't want "clinic" in the name because in South Florida the abortion clinics were being picketed and damaged by protesters. I needed to differentiate my practice from the abortion providers because that was not part of my practice.

3. One of my favorite memories of being a business owner is when I walked into the office and found my office manager holding onto the fire marshall (who was on a step stool) as he was changing the light bulb in one of our exit signs! She had developed such a wonderful relationship with the fire marshall that he didn't want to cite us for not being up to code, so he fixed the problem! Now, that is having friends in high places!

Resources

Blechman, BJ, and Levinson, JC: Guerrilla financing: Alternative techniques to finance any small business. Houghton Mifflin, Boston, 1992.

The Capitol Connection: *www.capitolconnection.com.*

Chesanow, N: Save thousands a year on medical supplies. Medical Economics Magazine: *www.pdr.net/memag/public.htm?path=docs/050800/article3.html.*

CLIA Application: *www.hcfa.gov/medicaid/clia/cliaapp.htm.*

Evanson, DR: Where to go when the bank says no: Alternatives for financing your business. Bloomberg Press, Princeton, 1988,

Federal Identification Number Application: *www.irs.ustreas.gov/prod/forms-pubs/.*

Grandinetti, DA: How location can make or break your practice. Medical Economics Magazine: *www.pdr.net/memag/public.htm?path=docs/061900/article4.html.*

Knopper, M: Your papers, please? A look into PA practice agreements and NP protocols. Clinician News 5, 6, 2001.

Lister, K: Finding Money: The Small Business Guide to Financing. John Wiley & Sons, New York, 1995.

LiveCapital Corporate: *www.livecapital.com/getfinancing.html.*

Location of local CLIA office: *www.hcfa.gov/medicaid/clia/ssa-map.htm.*

Narcotics license information: *www.deadiversion.usdoj.gov/drugreg/process.htm.*

National Association of Women Business Owners (NAWBO): *www.nawbo.org www.sba.gov.*

OSHA Standards: *www.osha.gov/.*

Provider performed microscopy information: *www.phppo.cdc.gov/clia/ppm.asp.*

Smith, R, and Edwards, MJ: The Internet for Physicians. Springer Verlag, New York, 2001.

NOTES

Chapter 5

Collaborative Relationships: How Do I Develop This Relationship?

" Coming together is the beginning; keeping together is progress; working together is success "

Henry Ford

In many states, a collaborative or supervisory relationship with a physician is required to practice as a nurse practitioner. Some people believe this requirement is restrictive and the requirement should be removed, but I believe the collaborative relationship can be the best and most important relationship in your career. If you are required to create this relationship, you can make it work well for you as well as for your physician. This is a relationship that is well worth developing and nurturing. Your collaborative physician can be your best teacher and ally.

DEFINITION OF COLLABORATION

There are many definitions available for the word *collaboration.* Basically, it is defined in *Webster's New World Dictionary and Thesaurus* as "the process of working together," implying shared planning and action over time. Collaboration involves working together to find solutions when both individuals' concerns are recognized and important concerns are not compromised.

The federal government, in the Medicare rules, has addressed collaborative relationships for nurse practitioners. The federal rules provide clear guidelines on collaboration. The rules state that services provided by a nurse practitioner or clinical nurse specialist must be provided in collaboration with a physician in accordance with state law in order to qualify for coverage. These rules recognize that state laws on nurse practitioner and clinical nurse specialist practice differ in their approach to collaboration.

> *Collaboration is a process in which a nurse practitioner [or clinical nurse specialist] works with one or more physicians to deliver health care services within the scope of the practitioner's expertise, with medical direction and appropriate supervision as provided for in jointly developed guidelines or other mechanisms as provided for by the law of the State in which the services are performed (42 CFR Section 410.75 (C)(3)(I); [emphasis added]).*

The federal rules defer to state requirements for collaboration. These rules and requirements can change—so be sure to keep current with your state and federal laws. The American Academy of Nurse Practitioners and the American College of Nurse Practitioners post the changes in their newsletters. If you are not a member of one or both organizations, you should be. Not only are you kept up to date on the changes in the laws and regulations but also these organizations lobby for positive changes for all nurse practitioners. Your local and state nurse practitioner organizations may also be very helpful in this area.

SELECTING A COLLABORATING PHYSICIAN

It is often said that a business partnership is like a marriage, and in both relationships large dollops of chemistry and luck are needed to keep things together. Selecting a collaborating physician is something you should do with a lot of thought and discussion. It is to your benefit to search for a physician who understands and respects the role of the nurse practitioner.

If you do not have a potential physician to approach for this relationship, ask around. Not only is it important to find a good physician to work with, it is also important to find out who to steer clear of. Ask other nurse practitioners. Go to a meeting with the local nurse practitioners for referrals. They may know physicians who are willing to work with nurse practitioners. Nurses at the local hospital may be able to refer you to nurse practitioner–friendly physicians.

Be prepared before you set up a meeting to interview a physician. Investigate and learn your state laws. Be able to answer questions regarding the regulations of your practice. Have a clear outline of what you will require from him or her. If you have prepared a management protocol, have a copy ready to hand over, along with your current curriculum vitae or resume. If you have not prepared a protocol, you may want to simply write out what type of patients you plan on seeing, what special procedures you will be performing, and what diagnostic tests you may be ordering. You want your collaborating physician to have a clear understanding of your practice before you agree to work together. Be prepared to answer questions. Do not be defensive; this is a time for education for the both of you. Listening to the physician during this interview is very important. Inattention can lead to miscommunication. Take notes to help you remember what you have discussed and agreed upon.

Topics to discuss when interviewing a potential collaborative physician include:

- Medical training
- Past experiences with nurse practitioners
- Availability for consultations
- Willingness to teach
- Limitations on your practice
- Handling of vacations

While you are interviewing your prospective collaborative physician, assess your level of comfort in conversation. If you are intimidated or uncomfortable while asking questions, you could be setting yourself up for failure. Identify your practice style and look for a physician with similar preferences. If you are an aggressive, cutting-edge practitioner, you may not work well with someone who uses a more conservative approach. Too many differences may foster discord. Finding someone with your same approach to patient care is very important. Depending on your situation, you may want to suggest working together for a designated time to really learn each other's treatment style and to become comfortable with your working relationship. Working together for a time could be especially helpful if you do not know each other well.

It is imperative for you to develop a good rapport with this person who is so important to your professional success. Malpractice history of your potential collaborative physician is another area you may want to investigate on your own. You may be able to access this information over the Internet or through the state regulatory board for physicians. Attaching your professional reputation to a physician is not something to take lightly. Check out the physician to make sure he or she is someone with whom you want to be associated.

COMPENSATION FOR YOUR COLLABORATING PHYSICIAN

There are many ways to approach compensation. Ideally, you would find a way for your relationship to benefit you both so that you do not have to pay him or her. When you are first starting your practice, there will be time when you are not seeing patients—maybe you could work for your collaborating physician a couple of days (or half days) during the week to lighten his or her load. You can use this as a learning experience as well. Maybe you could help cover after-hours emergency calls. Through your conversation during the interview, you may be able to identify a way to make things easier for the physician, which, in turn, may make negotiations easier for you.

Some nurse practitioners in independent practice pay their collaborating physician up to $1,000 per month. Some base the payments on a certain number of charts reviewed (e.g., 10 charts per month at $25 per chart). Some even base the payment on a percentage of their income.

Remember, some physicians may agree to work with you without compensation. However, you may want to offer to refer some patients to them. You want to keep your physician happy with your relationship. It should be beneficial to you both.

DEVELOPING AND NURTURING THE RELATIONSHIP

This is a relationship that should be based on mutual respect. If one of the parties involved does not respect the other, there is little hope for a successful relationship. The literature indicates that collaboration between nurses and physicians has become more sophisticated as these relationships have become collegial in nature and as nurses have become assertive, autonomous, and accountable.[1]

Nurses and physicians in collaborative relationships may want to think about their interprofessional communication styles—how they approach conflict resolution, clinical interaction, use of humor, and negotiation skills. Tradition, professionalism, concerns about practice boundaries, and competition continue to be obstacles to collaborative practice for some. They do not have to be obstacles for you.

Work at making your collaborative relationship the best that it can be. Develop a friendship and a collegial relationship. Trust on both sides of the relationship will come with time and experience. You can both grow and benefit from this relationship—nurture it!

SCOPE OF PRACTICE

The *scope of practice* for nurse practitioners is defined by the laws and rules of the state in which the nurse practitioner provides services. For more information on whether a service falls within the nurse practitioner's scope of practice, consult the state agency that regulates nurse practitioner practice (Table 5–1). These agencies are the ones to interpret the state's practice laws and resolve these questions. Again, your state and local nurse practitioner organizations may be helpful in this area.

Defining and following your scope of practice is your responsibility as a professional nurse practitioner. The American Nurses Publishing has produced an excellent resource, *Scope and Standards of Advanced Practice Registered Nursing,* which clearly defines both standards of care and professional performance.

Table 5–1	State Regulatory Agencies for Nurse Practitioner Practice

Alabama Board of Nursing RSA Plaza, Suite 250 770 Washington Ave. Montgomery, AL 36130-3900	Phone: 334-242-4060 Fax: 334-242-4360 Website: *www.abn.state.al.us*
Alaska Board of Nursing 3601 C St., Suite 722 Anchorage, AK 99503	Phone: 907-269-8161 Fax: 907-269-8196 Website: *www.dced.state.ak.us*
Arizona State Board of Nursing 1651 E. Morten Ave., Suite 210 Phoenix, AZ 85020	Phone: 602-331-8111 Fax: 602-906-9365 Website: *www.azboardofnursing.org/*
Arkansas State Board of Nursing University Tower Building 1123 S. University, Suite 800 Little Rock, AR 72204	Phone: 501-686-2700 Fax: 501-686-2714 Website: *www.state.ar.us/nurse*
California Board of Registered Nursing 400 R St., Suite. 4030 Sacramento, CA 95814-6239	Phone: 916-322-3350 Fax: 916-327-4402 Website: *www.rn.ca.gov*
Colorado Board of Nursing 1560 Broadway, Suite 880 Denver, CO 80202	Phone: 303-894-2430 Fax: 303-894-2821 Website: *www.dora.state.co.us/nursing/*
Connecticut Board of Examiners for Nursing Division of Health Systems Regulation 410 Capitol Ave., MS# 13ADJ P.O. Box 340308 Hartford, CT 06134-0328	Phone: 860-509-7624 Fax: 860-509-7553 Website: *http://www.state.ct.us/dph/*
Delaware Board of Nursing Cannon Building, Suite 203 861 Silver Lake Blvd. Dover, DE 19904	Phone: 302-739-4522 Fax: 302-739-2711
District of Columbia Board of Nursing Department of Health 825 N. Capitol St., N.E., 2nd Floor, Room 2224 Washington, DC 20002	Phone: 202-442-4778 Fax: 202-442-9431
Florida Board of Nursing 4080 Woodcock Drive, Suite 202 Jacksonville, FL 32207	Phone: 904-858-6940 Fax: 904-858-6964 Website: *http://www.doh.state.fl.us/mqa/nursing/rnhome.htm*
Georgia Board of Nursing 237 Coliseum Drive Macon, GA 31217-3858	Phone: 912-207-1640 Fax: 912-207-1660 Website: *http://www.sos.state.ga.us/ebd-rn/*
Hawaii Board of Nursing Professional and Vocational Licensing Division P.O. Box 3469 Honolulu, HI 96801	Phone: 808-586-3000 Fax: 808-586-2689 Website: *http://www.state.hi.us/dcca/pvloffline/*
Idaho Board of Nursing 280 N. 8th St., Suite 210 P.O. Box 83720 Boise, ID 83720	Phone: 208-334-3110 Fax: 208-334-3262 Website: *http://www.state.id.us/ibn/ibnhome.htm*
Illinois Department of Professional Regulation James R. Thompson Center 100 West Randolph, Suite 9-300 Chicago, IL 60601	Phone: 312-814-2715 Fax: 312-814-3145 Website: *http://www.dpr.state.il.us/*
Indiana State Board of Nursing Health Professions Bureau 402 W. Washington St., Room W041 Indianapolis, IN 46204	Phone: 317-232-2960 Fax: 317-233-4236 Website: *http://www.state.in.us/hpb/isbn/*

Table 5-1	State Regulatory Agencies for Nurse Practitioner Practice *[Continued]*
Iowa Board of Nursing River Point Business Park 400 S.W. 8th St. Suite B Des Moines, IA 50309-4685	Phone: 515-281-3255 Fax: 515-281-4825 Website: *http://www.state.ia.us/government/nursing/*
Kansas State Board of Nursing Landon State Office Building 900 S.W. Jackson, Suite 551-S Topeka, KS 66612	Phone: 785-296-4929 Fax: 785-296-3929 Website: *http://www.state.ia.us/government/nursing/*
Kentucky Board of Nursing 312 Whittington Parkway, Suite 300 Louisville, KY 40222	Phone: 502-329-7000 Fax:502-329-7011 Website: *http://www.kbn.state.ky.us/*
Louisiana State Board of Nursing 3510 N. Causeway Boulevard, Suite 501 Metairie, LA 70003	Phone: 504-838-5332 Fax:504-838-5349 Website: *http://www.lsbn.state.la.us/*
Maine State Board of Nursing 158 State House Station Augusta, ME 04333	Phone: 207-287-1133 Fax: 207-287-1149 Website: *www.state.me.us/nursing*
Maryland Board of Nursing 4140 Patterson Ave. Baltimore, MD 21215	Phone: 410-585-1900 Fax: 410-358-3530 Website: *http://dh,hld.dhmn.state.md.us/mbn*
Massachusetts Board of Registration In Nursing Commonwealth of Massachusetts 239 Causeway St. Boston, MA 02114	Phone: 617-727-9961 Fax: 617-727-1630 Website: *www.state.ma.us/reg/*
Michigan CIS/Office of Health Services Ottawa Towers North 611 W. Ottawa, 4th Floor Lansing, MI 48933	Phone: 517-373-9102 Fax: 517-373-2179 Website: *www.cis.state.mi.us*
Minnesota Board of Nursing 2829 University Ave. SE Suite 500 Minneapolis, MN 55414	Phone: 612-617-2270 Fax: 612-617-2190 Website: *www.nursingboard.state.mn.us/*
Mississippi Board of Nursing 1935 Lakeland Drive, Suite B Jackson, MS 39216	Phone: 601-987-4188 Fax: 601-364-2352 Website: *www.msbn.state.ms.us/*
Missouri State Board of Nursing 3605 Missouri Blvd. P.O. Box 656 Jefferson City, MO 65102-0656	Phone: 573-751-0681 Fax: 573-751-0075 Website: *www.ecodev.state.mo.us*
Montana State Board of Nursing 301 South Park Helena, MT 59620-0513	Phone: 406-444-2071 Fax: 406-841-2343 Website: *www.com.state.mo.us*
Nebraska Health and Human Services System Dept. of Regulation and Licensure, Nursing Section 301 Centennial Mall South, P.O. Box 94986 Lincoln, NE 68509-4986	Phone: 402-471-4376 Fax: 402-471-3577 Website: *www.hhs.state.ne.us*
Nevada State Board of Nursing 1755 East Plumb Lane, Suite 260 Reno, NV 89502	Phone: 775-688-2620 Fax: 775-688-2628 Website: *www.nursingboard.state.nv.us*
New Hampshire Board of Nursing 78 Regional Drive, BLDG B P.O. Box 3898 Concord, NH 03302	Phone: 603-271-2323 Fax: 603-271-6605 Website: *www.state.nh.us*

[Continued]

Table 5-1	State Regulatory Agencies for Nurse Practitioner Practice *[Continued]*

New Jersey Board of Nursing 124 Halsey St., 6th Floor P.O. Box 45010 Newark, NJ 07101	Phone: 973-504-6586 Fax: 973-648-3481 Website: *www.state.nj.us*
New Mexico Board of Nursing 4206 Louisiana Boulevard, NE Suite A Albuquerque, NM 87109	Phone: 505-841-8340 Fax: 505-841-8347 Website: *www.state.nm.us*
New York State Board of Nursing 89 Washington Ave. Education Bldg. 2nd Floor West Wing Albany, NY 12234	Phone: 518-473-6999 Fax: 518-474-3706 Website: *www.nysed.gov/prof/nurse.htm*
North Carolina Board of Nursing 3724 National Drive, Suite 201 Raleigh, NC 27612	Phone: 919-782-3211 Fax: 919-781-9461 Website: *www.ncbon.com*
North Dakota Board of Nursing 919 South 7th St., Suite 504 Bismarck, ND 58504	Phone: 701-328-9777 Fax: 701-328-9785 Website: *www.ndbon.org*
Ohio Board of Nursing 17 South High St., Suite 400 Columbus, OH 43215-3413	Phone: 614-466-3947 Fax: 614-466-0388 Website: *www.state.oh.us/nurse*
Oklahoma Board of Nursing 2915 N. Classen Boulevard, Suite 524 Oklahoma City, OK 73106	Phone: 405-962-1800 Fax: 405-962-1821
Oregon State Board of Nursing 800 NE Oregon St., Box 25 Suite 465 Portland, OR 97232	Phone: 503-731-4745 Fax: 503-731-4755 Website: *www.osbn.state.or.us*
Pennsylvania State Board of Nursing 124 Pine St. P.O. Box 2649 Harrisburg, PA 17101	Phone: 717-783-7142 Fax: 717-783-0822 Website: *www.dos.state.pa.us/bpoa/nurbd/mainpage.htm*
Commonwealth of Puerto Rico Board of Nurse Examiners 800 Roberto H. Todd Ave. Room 202, Stop 18 Santurce, PR 00908	Phone: 787-725-8161 Fax: 787-725-7903
Rhode Island Board of Nurse Registration and Nursing Education 105 Cannon Building Three Capitol Hill Providence, RI 02908	Phone: 401-222-5700 Fax: 401-222-3352 Website: *www.health.sgtate.ri.us*
South Carolina State Board of Nursing 110 Centerview Drive Suite 202 Columbia, SC 29210	Phone: 803-896-4550 Fax: 803-896-4525 Website: *www.llr.state.sc.us/pol/nursing*
South Dakota Board of Nursing 4300 South Louise Ave., Ste C-1 Sioux Falls, SD 57106-3124	Phone: 605-362-2760 Fax: 605-362-2768 Website: *www.state.sd.us/dcr/nursing*
Tennessee State Board of Nursing 426 Fifth Ave. North 1st Floor—Cordell Hull Building Nashville, TN 37247	Phone: 615-532-5166 Fax: 615-741-7899 Website: *http://170.142.76.180/bmf-bin/bmf*
Texas Board of Nurse Examiners 333 Guadalupe, Suite 3-460 Austin, TX 78701	Phone: 512-305-7400 Fax: 512-305-7401 Website: *www.bne.state.tx.us/*

Table 5-1	State Regulatory Agencies for Nurse Practitioner Practice *[Continued]*
Utah State Board of Nursing Heber M. Wells Bldg., 4th Floor 160 East 300 South Salt Lake City, UT 84111	Phone: 801-530-6628 Fax: 801-530-6511 Website: *http://www.commerce.state.ut.us/*
Vermont State Board of Nursing 109 State St. Montpelier, VT 05609-1106	Phone: 802-828-2396 Fax: 802-828-2484 Website: *www.vtprofessionals.org/nurses*
Virgin Islands Board of Nurse Licensure Veterans Drive Station St. Thomas, VI 00803	Phone: 340-776-7397 Fax: 340-777-4003
Virginia Board of Nursing 6606 W. Broad St., 4th Floor Richmond, VA 23230	Phone: 804-662-9909 Fax: 804-662-9512 Website: *http://www.dhp.state.va.us/*
Washington State Nursing Care Quality Assurance Commission Department of Health 1300 Quince St. SE Olympia, WA 98504-7864	Phone: 360-236-4740 Fax: 360-236-4738 Website: *www.doh.wa.gov/nursing/*
West Virginia Board of Examiners for Registered Professional Nurses 101 Dee Drive Charleston, WV 25311	Phone: 304-558-3596 Fax: 304-558-3666 Website: *www.state.wv.us/nurses*
Wisconsin Department of Regulation & Licensing 1400 E. Washington Ave. P.O. Box 8935 Madison, WI 53708	Phone: 608-266-0145 Fax: 608-261-7083 Website: http://www.drl.state.wi.us/
Wyoming State Board of Nursing 2020 Carey Ave., Suite 110 Cheyenne, WY 82002	Phone: 307-777-7601 Fax: 307-777-3519 Website: http://nursing.state.wy.us/

COLLABORATING PHYSICIAN'S LIABILITY

This is an area that is difficult to understand unless you become involved in a malpractice lawsuit. Historically, some physicians have been held liable for the negligent acts of nurse practitioners with whom they have a collaborative relationship. Every case is different; the physician may or may not be attached to the lawsuit depending on his or her involvement in the case. Hopefully you will not have to learn about this first hand. As long as the laws in your state require a supervisory or collaborative relationship, the collaborating or supervising physician may be exposed to potential lawsuits.

REFERRALS AND CONSULTATIONS

The importance of building networks with local providers should not be ignored. Having a good list of providers to refer to in every specialty is critical. You want to be able to call on these providers as needed and get the attention for your patients as needed. You may also enjoy referrals from these providers over time. Once they learn to trust your clinical judgment and you demonstrate your ability to work within your scope of practice, you may be considered one of their peers. This relationship may take time to build. These referral providers can be allies who can assist you in an emergency. It is also important to find out who to stay away from. You may be held liable for the actions of the providers you refer to.

You should be prepared before you make a telephone call for a consultation or to refer a patient. Have all of the patient's information in front of you and be prepared to answer questions. Communicate clearly and concisely. Be polite and respectful of the physician's time. Referral and consultation relationships are relationships to treasure and nurture.

Many times your patients will ask you for a referral to a specialty physician or nurse practitioner. Develop and print a list of local providers and their specialty and contact information. This is a time-saver when you make referrals. Include up to three providers in each specialty, since many insurance companies dictate whom the patients can see for their health care.

PRACTICE COVERAGE

Depending on your type of practice, you may need to make arrangements for when you are out of town or unavailable. Investigate how providers in your specialty and community handle coverage for their offices. You may want to hire a nurse practitioner or physician to see patients in your office if you will be gone for an extended amount of time. If you do hire someone, be prepared to pay them, handle payroll deductions, and follow the laws as far as written protocols and so forth. You may just have your patients call the providers of your choice to be seen at the provider's office. Communicate with your collaborating physician; see what he or she can do for you while you are on vacation. Really think this through so you can relax during your time away. You need to have the confidence that your patients will be receiving quality care while you are away.

SUGGESTIONS AND TIPS FROM WOMEN'S HEALTH WATCH, INC.

- The collaborating physicians for Women's Health Watch, Inc., have been fantastic. When developing the practice, the collaborating physician was very supportive. I worked for him two half-days a week, which freed him up to perform more surgeries and resulted in a substantial increase in revenues for his practice. In return, besides per diem payment, he signed my management protocol and supported me in all of my projects. In turn, the money I was paid for the two half-days of work paid my office manager's salary! I really can't think of any way the relationship could have been better.

■ Developing a method for regular communication with your collaborating physician is very important. We had a notepad that was on the desk we shared and we were able to write notes and questions to each other. Because we didn't see patients at the same time in that office, it was a nice way to ask questions and share information without disturbing each other during office hours.

PERSONAL ANECDOTES

1. I have been very fortunate with my relationships with my collaborating physicians. I chose physicians who were well versed in the role of the nurse practitioner and were very supportive. What a comfort it is to have someone working with you who truly believes in you and your ability to provide quality health care.

2. It was a pleasant surprise to find that patients were being referred to me from local physicians and clinics. Physicians appreciate referrals just as you do. They may want to reciprocate and develop a working relationship with you.

Resources

Allen, DW, et al: Employment contracts, negotiation strategies, and the nurse practitioner. The 2001 Sourcebook for Advanced Practice Nurses 4:12–17, 2001.

Burchell, RC, et al: Some considerations for implementing collaborative practice. Am J Med 74:9–13, 1983.

Collins-Bride, GM, and Saxe, JM: Nurse practitioner/physician collaborative practice: Clinical guidelines. UCSF Nursing Press, San Francisco, 1999.

Neufeldt, V, and Sparks, AN (eds): Webster's New World Dictionary: Compact School Office Edition. New York: Prentice-Hall, 1989.

Scope and Standards of Advanced Practice Registered Nursing. American Nurses Publishing, Washington, DC, 1996.

Washington Word. Am Coll Nurse Pract (2000, September) 3:1–2, 2001.

Weiss, S, and Davis, HP: Validity and reliability of the collaborative practice scales. Nursing Res 34:229–305, 1985.

Reference

1. Taylor-Seehafer, M: Nurse-physician collaboration. J Am Acad Nurse Pract 10:387–391, 1998.

N O T E S

Chapter 6

Patient Payments: How Much Do I Charge and How Do I Collect?

" Money is the symbol of duty. It is the sacrament of having done for mankind that which mankind wanted "

Samuel Butler

This is a critical area in which you need to consider all aspects of patient payments, including setting office policy, defining your procedures, and deciding what to charge for every potential service and product you will provide. You will need to learn about billing, reimbursement, and the laws that govern Medicaid and Medicare payments. It may all seem overwhelming. Don't let it be; just take it one step at a time.

PAYMENT FOR SERVICES

Unless you are starting a free clinic under a grant or you have found some other magical source that will pay your bills, you will need to design the payment system for your office. Because you have already defined your target market (patient description), you should have an idea of how you plan to be paid. Types of payment to consider include the following:

- Cash (always good!)
- Checks (not always good!)
- Credit cards
- Medicaid
- Medicare
- HMO
- Indemnity insurance

Once you define which types of payment you will accept, design appropriate collection procedures. It is critical that you have a responsible and trustworthy person handling all payments! There are far too many stories about health-care providers being swindled by their office staff. Do not be naive. Design checks and balances for you, so you can have the knowledge and confidence that your patient income is being handled correctly. Remember, no one can walk on you if you don't lie down to let them! Be in control. It is tempting as a provider to separate yourself from the finances of your practice. If you do, you may end up without a practice. This is a business, you are the owner, and you need to take the responsibility of knowing exactly what payment is coming in and what you are paying out.

SETTING YOUR FEES

Defining your practice will help you set your fees. Do you picture your practice as a clinic? A posh private practice? Someplace between the two? You need to identify what the customary charges are for initial visits and some procedures in your community before you set your fees. Start by listing all of the different types of office visits and procedures you plan on providing (Fig. 6–1).

It would be ideal if you were able to have detailed lists of charges from a local doctor, clinic, and/or nurse practitioner before you start arbitrarily assigning charges for your services. You can always change them later. For the procedures, be sure to account for the costs of the supplies and equipment needed. If you are going to be giving shots or immunizations, be sure to calculate the cost per shot. Laboratory fees are usually triple or quadruple what the laboratory is charging to process the specimen. You need to make sure your prices are not too high and not too low. Simple telephone calls to area providers are a good way to learn what is being charged for specific tests and procedures. Cash paying patients may be calling your office for your fees. Check your fees on a regular basis to ensure that you are maximizing your revenues.

Once you have established your fee schedule, keep current copies handy for quick reference. To properly charge patients for services rendered, office personnel must have current fee schedules that are accurate and complete.

SUPERBILL

The *superbill* is the basic receipt that is given to the patient. It should include all of the information that is required by insurance companies for reimbursement. By including this information, the number of telephone calls from insurance carriers to your office will be reduced and payment will be expedited. The key components of the superbill include:

- Name of the practice
- Address

Figure 6-1	Setting Your Fees

Visit/Procedure	MD	NP	Clinic	Your Office
Eg: Initial Visit	$150	$75	$55	$75
Re-Visit	$50	$35	$20	$40

- Telephone and Fax numbers
- Tax ID number
- Provider's name and credentials
- Patient's name (clearly written)
- Date of service
- All the procedures and visits with the appropriate codes
- All laboratory tests with appropriate codes
- All potential diagnoses with the appropriate codes
- Method of payment
- Total due
- Total paid
- Balance due

Look at the sample superbill provided (Fig 6–2). You may want to leave a few blank lines under the procedure, laboratory, and diagnosis sections for the unexpected. This can be designed by you and printed at a local printer on plain white paper. After you are finished with your patient's visit, mark off the appropriate visit, diagnosis, and procedures performed on the superbill. If your diagnosis or procedure is not on your printed superbill, take the time immediately to look up the correct codes. Be sure to give every patient a copy of a correct and complete superbill to take home. After you have completed the superbill, simply make a copy for the patient. You may want to reevaluate the form after a few months of practice. You may want to add or change certain items. You will also need to know that the codes you are using are the correct codes for your patients.

SELF PAY (OR FEE-FOR-SERVICE)

Patients who pay for their health care out of their own pockets may be rare in your community, or they may be the majority. You may be surprised at how many self-paying patients your practice will attract. The term "fee-for-service" is the traditional health-care payment system in which the patient is charged according to a set fee schedule for each visit and procedure. When patients call to schedule a visit, you should tell them how much the visit will be and that if any other testing is necessary you will discuss the charges with them before proceeding. You want them to have a realistic idea of how much money to bring. Also tell them what types of payment you accept, for example, that you do not accept checks but that you do take certain credit cards. Have a section on the patient information sheet for the patients to indicate how they plan to pay for their visit. Make sure you have a cash drawer that locks. Only the person handling the cash should be allowed in that drawer. Prepare for cash-paying patients by having smaller bills for change.

Figure 6-2 Sample Superbill

WOMEN'S HEALTH WATCH, INC.

TAX ID # XX-XXXXXXX
Nurse Practioner Name

4540 N. Federal Hwy.
Ft. Lauderdale, FL 33308
(954) 776-1500   FAX (954) 776-1501

PATIENT'S NAME _____

DATE OF SERVICE _____   ARNP _____

PROCEDURE
____	99203	Initial Visit
____	W9760	AV Annual Visit
____	99212	Revisit
____	W9851	Supply Visit
____	W9850	CV Counseling Visit
____	17110	Condyloma Destruction
____	J1055	DP Injection
____	57170	Diaphragm Fitting
____	58300	IUD Insertion
____	58301	IUD Removal
____	11975	Norplant Insertion
____	W9854	Norplant Kit
____	11976	Norplant Removal
____	57605	Endometrial Biopsy
____	57160	Pessary Insertion
____	57454	Colposcopy with BX
____	58999	Removal of Foreign Body
____	57511	Cryo Surgery-Cervix
____	10060	Incision & Drainage-Cyst
____	76856	Pelvic Ultrasound
____	87210	Wet Smear
____	90782	Injection
____	____	_____
____	____	_____
____	____	_____

LABS
____	80019	Chem25/CBC
____	80061	Coronary Risk
____	87087	Culture (misc)
____	83001	FSH
____	85018	Hemoglobin
____	87250	Herpes Culture
____	80091	Hyperthyroid Profile
____	80092	Hypothyroid Profile
____	80178	Lithium Level
____	88155	Pap Smear
____	84703	Pregnancy Test—Serum
____	81025	Pregnancy Test—Urine
____	84146	Prolactin—Serum
____	86580	TB Skin Test
____	87060	Throat Culture
____	81000	Urinalysis
____	87066	Urine Culture
____	57110	Chlamydia
____	87063	Gonorrhea
____	86659	HIV
____	86592	RPR
____	____	_____

DIAGNOSIS
____	Abnormal Pap Smear	795.0
____	Amenorrhea	626.0
____	Anemia	285.9
____	Bartholin Cyst	516.2
____	Breast Lump/Cyst	611.72
____	Cervical Polyp	622.7
____	Chlamydia	079.0
____	Condyloma	091.3
____	Constipation	564.0
____	Counseling (Test Results)	V65.4
____	Depo Provera	V25.49
____	External Hemorrhoid	455.3
____	Folliculitis	704.8
____	Foreign Body	939.2
____	Herpes	054.9
____	Hyperlipidemia	272.4
____	Hypertension	401.9
____	IUD	V25.42
____	Irregular Menses	625.4
____	Lymphadenopahy	785.6
____	Menopausal Syndrome	627.2
____	Metrorrhagia	626.6
____	Molluscum Contagiosum	078.0
____	Obesity	278.0
____	Otitis Media	382.0
____	Ovarian Cyst	620.2
____	Pelvic Mass	789.3
____	Pelvic Pain	625.8
____	PID	614.9
____	PMS	625.4
____	Polymenorrhea (Ex M)	626.2
____	Post Partum F/U	V24.2
____	Pregnancy	V22.2
____	Sinusitis	473.9
____	Skin Lesion	709.9
____	STD	099.0
____	Thyroid Enlarged	240.9
____	Tobacco Dependency	305.1
____	Trichomonas	131.00
____	URI	465.9
____	UTI	599.9
____	Uterine Fibroid	218.9
____	Vaginitis/Vulvo	616.10
____	Well Woman	V72.3
____	Contraception	V25.01
____	_____	____

Method of Payment _____

Total $ _____

Paid $ _____

Balance $ _____

Develop a check policy and post it in the office. There are services that will guarantee checks, but, of course, they charge a fee. One way to reduce the number of bad checks received is to only accept checks from established patients—not first time patients. Your bank will provide you with a rubber stamp to stamp the back of the check with your account name and number before depositing it. If a check is returned to you for insufficient funds, you will be charged a fee by your bank. Decide how much over that charge you will be charging your patient for the inconvenience. When speaking with them, you can ask whether they have a credit card and take the number over the phone to charge them the amount you decided upon plus what they owe you.

Some people use credit cards for all of their expenses. Having the capability of accepting credit cards could potentially increase your revenues significantly. That doesn't mean you have to accept all cards, just the ones you want to accept. You can either buy or lease the terminal, which simply hooks up to a telephone line and a power outlet. Shop around to find the best rates. You may want to ask around to find a company that is easy to work with and has a good reputation—your banking representative may have some suggestions.

Many companies provide credit card service (Merchant Services, PayNet, Bank of America, to name a few). The rate they charge for their services depends on your projected volume. After 6 months or 1 year, you can ask the credit card service provider to reevaluate the rate, particularly if you are doing a lot of credit card business.

If, for some reason, a patient is unable to pay in full, document it on the superbill, give the patient a copy, and ask him or her when and how they plan on paying. Suggest that the patient drop the payment in the mail slot after hours, or even give out a pre-addressed envelope. This is really a practice to discourage. A sign should be posted in the waiting area indicating that you expect payment at the time of service.

Accounts receivable and collection systems are used by the provider to record and track accounts receivable and are critical to the collection process.

INSURERS

Dealing with insurers could be an entire book by itself. Indemnity insurers are insurance companies that pay for the medical care of the insured, but they do not provide the health-care service. Providers are paid for each visit and procedure. To receive payment, the provider must submit a detailed billing form. The CMS Form 1500 is the standard billing form (Fig. 6–3).

This form is used for insurance companies, Medicare, and Medicaid. These forms can be purchased from the American Medical Association, 515 N. State Street, Chicago, IL 60610, or from your medical stationery supply company, or they can be downloaded from the Website at Center for Medicare and Medicaid Services at *http://www.hcfa.gov/medicare/edi/cms1500.pdf*.

Figure 6–3 Health Insurance Claim Form

PLEASE DO NOT STAPLE IN THIS AREA

CARRIER

PICA **HEALTH INSURANCE CLAIM FORM** PICA

1. MEDICARE (Medicare #) MEDICAID (Medicaid #) CHAMPUS (Sponsor's SSN) CHAMPVA (VA File #) GROUP HEALTH PLAN (SSN or ID) FECA BLK LUNG (SSN) OTHER (ID)

1a. INSURED'S I.D. NUMBER (FOR PROGRAM IN ITEM 1)

2. PATIENT'S NAME (Last Name, First Name, Middle Initial)

3. PATIENT'S BIRTH DATE MM DD YY SEX M F

4. INSURED'S NAME (Last Name, First Name, Middle Initial)

5. PATIENT'S ADDRESS (No., Street)

CITY STATE

ZIP CODE TELEPHONE (Include Area Code) ( )

6. PATIENT RELATIONSHIP TO INSURED Self Spouse Child Other

7. INSURED'S ADDRESS (No., Street)

CITY STATE

ZIP CODE TELEPHONE (INCLUDE AREA CODE) ( )

8. PATIENT STATUS Single Married Other Employed Full-Time Student Part-Time Student

9. OTHER INSURED'S NAME (Last Name, First Name, Middle Initial)

a. OTHER INSURED'S POLICY OR GROUP NUMBER

b. OTHER INSURED'S DATE OF BIRTH MM DD YY SEX M F

c. EMPLOYER'S NAME OR SCHOOL NAME

d. INSURANCE PLAN NAME OR PROGRAM NAME

10. IS PATIENT'S CONDITION RELATED TO:

a. EMPLOYMENT? (CURRENT OR PREVIOUS) YES NO

b. AUTO ACCIDENT? PLACE (State) YES NO

c. OTHER ACCIDENT? YES NO

10d. RESERVED FOR LOCAL USE

11. INSURED'S POLICY GROUP OR FECA NUMBER

a. INSURED'S DATE OF BIRTH MM DD YY SEX M F

b. EMPLOYER'S NAME OR SCHOOL NAME

c. INSURANCE PLAN NAME OR PROGRAM NAME

d. IS THERE ANOTHER HEALTH BENEFIT PLAN? YES NO *If yes*, return to and complete item 9 a-d.

READ BACK OF FORM BEFORE COMPLETING & SIGNING THIS FORM.

12. PATIENT'S OR AUTHORIZED PERSON'S SIGNATURE I authorize the release of any medical or other information necessary to process this claim. I also request payment of government benefits either to myself or to the party who accepts assignment below.

SIGNED ____ DATE ____

13. INSURED'S OR AUTHORIZED PERSON'S SIGNATURE I authorize payment of medical benefits to the undersigned physician or supplier for services described below.

SIGNED ____

PATIENT AND INSURED INFORMATION

14. DATE OF CURRENT: MM DD YY ILLNESS (First symptom) OR INJURY (Accident) OR PREGNANCY(LMP)

15. IF PATIENT HAS HAD SAME OR SIMILAR ILLNESS. GIVE FIRST DATE MM DD YY

16. DATES PATIENT UNABLE TO WORK IN CURRENT OCCUPATION FROM MM DD YY TO MM DD YY

17. NAME OF REFERRING PHYSICIAN OR OTHER SOURCE

17a. I.D. NUMBER OF REFERRING PHYSICIAN

18. HOSPITALIZATION DATES RELATED TO CURRENT SERVICES FROM MM DD YY TO MM DD YY

19. RESERVED FOR LOCAL USE

20. OUTSIDE LAB? YES NO $ CHARGES

21. DIAGNOSIS OR NATURE OF ILLNESS OR INJURY. (RELATE ITEMS 1,2,3 OR 4 TO ITEM 24E BY LINE)

1. ___ . __ 3. ___ . __

2. ___ . __ 4. ___ . __

22. MEDICAID RESUBMISSION CODE ORIGINAL REF. NO.

23. PRIOR AUTHORIZATION NUMBER

24. A DATE(S) OF SERVICE From MM DD YY To MM DD YY	B Place of Service	C Type of Service	D PROCEDURES, SERVICES, OR SUPPLIES (Explain Unusual Circumstances) CPT/HCPCS MODIFIER	E DIAGNOSIS CODE	F $ CHARGES	G DAYS OR UNITS	H EPSDT Family Plan	I EMG	J COB	K RESERVED FOR LOCAL USE
1										
2										
3										
4										
5										
6										

25. FEDERAL TAX I.D. NUMBER SSN EIN

26. PATIENT'S ACCOUNT NO.

27. ACCEPT ASSIGNMENT? (For govt. claims, see back) YES NO

28. TOTAL CHARGE $

29. AMOUNT PAID $

30. BALANCE DUE $

31. SIGNATURE OF PHYSICIAN OR SUPPLIER INCLUDING DEGREES OR CREDENTIALS (I certify that the statements on the reverse apply to this bill and are made a part thereof.)

SIGNED DATE

32. NAME AND ADDRESS OF FACILITY WHERE SERVICES WERE RENDERED (If other than home or office)

33. PHYSICIAN'S, SUPPLIER'S BILLING NAME, ADDRESS, ZIP CODE & PHONE #

PIN# GRP#

PHYSICIAN OR SUPPLIER INFORMATION

(APPROVED BY AMA COUNCIL ON MEDICAL SERVICE 8/88) ***PLEASE PRINT OR TYPE*** APPROVED OMB-0938-0008 FORM CMS-1500 (12-90), FORM RRB-1500, APPROVED OMB-1215-0055 FORM OWCP-1500, APPROVED OMB-0720-0001 (CHAMPUS)

Managed care companies differ from the indemnity insurers in that they not only pay for the medical care of the insured, but they also provide the health care for the insured. Managed care companies contract at reduced rates, basically in exchange for sending you clients without the cost of advertisement to you. Over the years, more and more nurse practitioners are being accepted onto the provider panels for managed care companies. Once you are accepted onto the panel and are designated as a *primary care provider,* you will receive a contract to provide care for their insured. You should be listed in the directory and receive reimbursement. Be prepared to provide written requests for authorization of continued service. Authorization codes must be provided on the CMS Form 1500 or the patient will be denied for the services—in other words, you won't get paid! As the *primary care provider,* you will have the full responsibility for the patient's primary care. Each company will have specific requirements regarding referrals, patient satisfaction, cost containment, and so on. With each contract, you must read through thoroughly to know what your responsibilities entail. The contract is a **contract.** Do not enter into the relationship lightly. Be sure you understand every element of the contract. It may be beneficial to find an attorney who can help you understand what you are signing. There are articles and books available specifically on negotiating contracts with managed care organizations.

Identify the HMO and insurance companies that are prominent in your community. These will be the first on your list when applying for provider status. If there are major industries in your community that use only a few insurance companies, it would be wise to contact them first.

MEDICARE

Medicare is a federal program, administered nationally by the Centers for Medicare and Medicaid Services (CMS, formerly the Health Care Finance Administration, HCFA), and is administered locally by Medicare carrier agencies. Medicare covers patients who are 65 years of age and older who have enrolled and pay premiums, as well as disabled individuals who qualify for Social Security disability payments and benefits. Medicare is divided into two parts. Medicare A covers hospitals, skilled nursing facilities, and some home health services. Medicare B covers services of physicians and other providers, outpatient hospital services, laboratory services, medical equipment, and additional home health expenses.

In 1997, the laws were changed to include nurse practitioners as providers for certain services. The first step in becoming a Medicare provider is to apply for provider status. To obtain an application (HCFA Form 855), contact your local Medicare Part B carrier for your region and request a provider enrollment application to become a Medicare provider or retrieve the application at *http://www.hcfa.gov/medicare/enrollment/forms/cms855i.pdf.* Medicare carriers are insurance companies that have contracted with the state to administer the program. Table 6–1 lists local Medicare Part B carriers. Once you receive the application, fill it out carefully and clearly.

Once you are approved to be a provider, your Medicare carrier in your region will issue you a PIN (provider identification number). The PIN is also referred to as your Medicare provider number. You must have a PIN to bill Medicare directly. Nurse practitioners are reimbursed at 85 percent of what they pay physicians for the same service. You will also receive a UPIN (unique physician identification number). If you are practicing at different sites, you will need to apply for a PIN for each site, whereas your UPIN remains constant.

An excellent resource for nurse practitioners is *Understanding Payment for Advanced Practice Nursing Services: Volume One: Medicare Reimbursement*, which is available through the American Nurses Association. This book goes into great detail on the requirements for application, enrolling, Medicare managed care, billing, claim denials, and fraud. This book also includes samples of several Medicare forms. This should be considered a required handbook for all nurse practitioners who are interested in providing services for Medicare patients. *Incident to* billing applies to nurse practitioners who are working for physicians. However, you may bill *incident to* for services provided by your staff following the same rules. Another resource you may find helpful in coding is the HCFA-produced *Evaluation and Management Documentation Guidelines*, which indicates the amount of documentation required for each of the five levels of evaluation and management visits. Nurse practitioners must base their choice of procedure code on the amount and complexity of evaluation and management services provided. If you are going to perform a service that is not covered by Medicare the patient must be informed.

Table 6–1	Medicare Part B State Carriers

Alabama

Medicare/Blue Cross-Blue Shield of Alabama
P.O. Box 830139
Birmingham, AL 35283-0139
205-981-4842

Alaska

Medicare/Noridian Mutual Insurance Company
4305 13th Ave., SW
Fargo, ND 58103
1-800-247-2267

Arizona

Medicare/ Noridian Mutual Insurance Company
4305 13th Ave., SW
Fargo, ND 58103
1-800-247-2267

Arkansas

Medicare/Arkansas Blue Cross-Blue Shield
601 Gaines St.
Little Rock, AK 72201
501-378-2250

[Continued]

Table 6-1	**Medicare Part B State Carriers** [Continued]

California

Medicare/Transamerica Occidental Life Insurance Company
Box 54905
Los Angeles, CA 90054-0905
1-800-675-2266
and
National Heritage Insurance Company
450 W. East Ave.
Chico, CA 95973
972-604-6251

Colorado

Medicare/Noridian Mutual Insurance Company
4305 13th Ave., SW
Fargo, ND 58103
1-800-247-2267

Connecticut

Medicare/MetraHealth Insurance Company
450 Columbus Boulevard-CT029-05AA
Hartford, CT 06103-1801
860-702-6667

Delaware

Blue Cross-Blue Shield of Texas
d.b.a. Trail Blazers Health Enterprises, Inc.
P.O. Box 660156
Dallas, TX 75266-0156
972-766-6900

District of Columbia

Blue Cross-Blue Shield of Texas
d.b.a. Trail Blazers Health Enterprises, Inc.
P.O. Box 660156
Dallas, TX 75266-0156
972-766-6900

Florida

Medicare/Blue Cross and Blue Shield of Florida, Inc.
P.O. Box 2078
Jacksonville, FL 32231-0048
1-800-333-7586

Georgia

Medicare/Blue Cross-Blue Shield of Alabama
P.O. Box 830139
Birmingham, AL 35283-0139
205-981-4842

Hawaii

Medicare/Noridian Mutual Insurance Company
4305 13th Ave., SW
Fargo, ND 58103
1-800-247-2267

Idaho

Medicare/Connecticut General Life Insurance Company
2 Vantage Way
Metro Exchange Bldg.
Nashville, TN 37228
615-782-4672

Illinois

Wisconsin Physicians Service Insurance Corporation
P.O. Box 1787
Madison, WI 53701
608-221-5084

| **Table 6-1** | **Medicare Part B State Carriers** *[Continued]* |

Indiana

Medicare Part B/AdminaStar Federal
P.O. Box 7073
Indianapolis, IN 46250
1-800-622-4792

Iowa

Medicare Part B/Noridian Mutual Insurance Company
4305 13th Ave., SW
Fargo, ND 58103
1-800-247-2267

Kansas

Medicare/Blue Cross-Blue Shield of Kansas, Inc.
P.O. Box 239
Topeka, KS 66601
1-800-432-3531

Kentucky

Medicare Part B/AdminaStar Federal, Inc.
P.O. Box 7073
Indianapolis, IN 46250
1-800-622-4792

Louisiana

Medicare/Arkansas Blue Cross-Blue Shield
601 Gaines St.
Little Rock, Arkansas 72201
1-800-462-9666

Maine

Medicare/National Heritage Insurance Company
450 W. East Ave.
Chico, CA 95973
972-604-6251

Maryland

Blue Cross-Blue Shield of Texas
d.b.a. Trail Blazers Health Enterprises, Inc.
P.O. Box 660156
Dallas, TX 75266-0156
972-766-1765

Massachusetts

Medicare/National Heritage Insurance Company
450 W. East Ave.
Chico, CA 95973
972-604-6251

Michigan

HCSC
Medicare Part B/Wisconsin Physicians Service Insurance Corporation
P.O. Box 8190
Madison, WI 53708
608-221-5084

Minnesota

Medicare/MetraHealth Insurance Company
450 Columbus Boulevard-CT029-05AA
Hartford, CT 06115-0450
860-702-6668

Mississippi

Medicare/MetraHealth Insurance Company
450 Columbus Boulevard-CT029-05AA
Hartford, CT 06115-0450
1-800-682-5417

[Continued]

Table 6-1	**Medicare Part B State Carriers** *[Continued]*

Missouri

Medicare/Blue Cross-Blue Shield of Kansas, Inc.
P.O. Box 239
Topeka, KS 66601
913-291-7000
and
Medicare/Arkansas Blue Cross-Blue Shield
601 Gaines St.
Little Rock, AK 72201
1-800-462-9666

Montana

Medicare/Blue Cross and Blue Shield of Montana, Inc.
P.O. Box 4310
Helena, MT 59604
1-800-332-3146

Nebraska

Medicare/Blue Cross-Blue Shield of Kansas, Inc.
P.O. Box 239
Topeka, KS 66601
785-291-4155

Nevada

Medicare Part B/Noridian Mutual Insurance Company
4305 13th Ave., SW
Fargo, ND 58103
1-800-247-2267

New Hampshire

Medicare/National Heritage Insurance Company
450 W. East Ave.
Chico, CA 95973
916-896-7025

New Jersey

Highmark, Inc.
d.b.a. Xact Medicare Services
P.O. Box 890065
Camp Hill, PA 17089
1-800-462-9306

New Mexico

Medicare/Arkansas Blue Cross-Blue Shield
601 Gaines St.
Little Rock, AK 72201
405-848-6257

New York

Medicare B/Empire Blue Cross and Blue Shield
P.O. Box 2280
New York, NY 10017
914-248-2852
and
Medicare/Group Health, Incorporated
P.O. Box 1608, Ansonia Station
New York, NY 10023
212-721-1770
and
BC/BS of Western New York
Upstate Medicare Division Part B
P.O. Box 5236
Binghamton, NY 13905-5236
1-800-252-6550

| **Table 6-1** | **Medicare Part B State Carriers** *[Continued]* |

North Carolina

Medicare/Connecticut General Life Insurance Company
2 Vantage Way
Metro Exchange Bldg.
Nashville, TN 37228
615-782-4525

North Dakota

Medicare Part B/Noridian Mutual Insurance Company
4305 13th Ave., SW
Fargo, ND 58103
1-800-247-2267

Ohio

Medicare/Nationwide Mutual Insurance Company
P.O. Box 16788
Columbus, OH 43216-6788
1-800-282-0530

Oklahoma

Medicare/Arkansas Blue Cross-Blue Shield
601 Gaines St.
Little Rock AK 72201
405-848-6257

Oregon

Medicare Part B/Noridian Mutual Insurance Company
4305 13th Ave., SW
Fargo, ND 58103
1-800-247-2267

Pennsylvania

Highmark, Incorporated
d.b.a. Xact Medicare Services
P.O. Box 890065
Camp Hill, PA 17089-0065
1-800-382-1274

Rhode Island

Medicare/Blue Cross and Blue Shield of Rhode Island
Inquiry Department
444 Westminster St.
Providence, RI 02903-3279
1-800-662-5170

South Carolina

Blue Cross and Blue Shield of South Carolina
Medicare Part B Operations
1-20 At Alphine Road
Columbia, SC 29219
1-800-868-2522

South Dakota

Medicare Part B/Noridian Mutual Insurance Company
4305 13th Ave., SW
Fargo, ND 58103
1-800-247-2267

Tennessee

Medicare/Connecticut General Life Insurance Company
2 Vantage Way
Metro Exchange Bldg.
Nashville, TN 37228
615-782-4484

[Continued]

Table 6-1   **Medicare Part B State Carriers** *[Continued]*

Texas

Blue Cross-Blue Shield of Texas
d.b.a. Trail Blazers Health Enterprises, Inc.
P.O. Box 660156
Dallas, TX 75266-0156
972-766-6900

Utah

Medicare/Blue Shield of Utah
P.O. Box 30269
Salt Lake City, Utah 84130-0269
1-800-426-3477

Vermont

Medicare/ National Heritage Insurance Company
450 W. East Ave.
Chico, CA 95973
916-896-7025

Virginia

MetraHealth Insurance Company
P.O. Box 26463
300 Arboretum Place
Richmond, VA 23236
804-327-2100

Washington

Medicare Part B/Noridian Mutual Insurance Company
4305 13th Ave., SW
Fargo, ND 58103
1-800-247-2267

West Virginia

Medicare/Nationwide Mutual Insurance Company
P.O. Box 16788
Columbus, OH 43216-6788
1-800-848-0106

Wisconsin

Wisconsin Medicare/WPS
Box 1787
Madison, WI 53701
1-800-828-2837

Wyoming

Medicare Part B/Noridian Mutual Insurance Company
4305 13th Ave., SW
Fargo, ND 58103
1-800-247-2267

Puerto Rico

Medicare Triple-S, Incorporated
P.O. Box 71391
San Juan, Puerto Rico 00936-1391
1-800-981-7015

Virgin Islands

Medicare Triple-S, Incorporated
P.O. Box 71391
San Juan, Puerto Rico 00936-1391
809-774-7915

More information is available at *www.hcfa.gov/medicare/incardir.htm*

MEDICAID

Medicaid is a federal program that is administered by the individual states. It was created for mothers and children who qualify on the basis of poverty. It is also for adults who are disabled for the short term—1 year or less—and who qualify on the basis of poverty. To apply for provider status with Medicaid, contact the state Medicaid agency (Table 6–2).

The provider relations department can provide an application. The reimbursement process varies by state. When speaking with the provider relations department, ask whether there is someone that specifically works with nurse practitioners; there may be such a liaison. It is beneficial to have a person you can call directly with questions or problems. Many states supply software that enables you to charge Medicaid directly online; they may also be able to directly deposit your check into your bank account. These systems can speed up the reimbursement process significantly. Be sure to read through all the materials given to you. You will be receiving updates. You need to stay on top of this information. If you are denied payment for a service you think should have been covered, contact your representative from the Medicaid office. Depending on the volume of Medicaid patients, you may or may not be reimbursed for a significant amount of money. However, every dollar counts when you are building your practice.

TERMS AND DEFINITIONS

The insurance business seems to have its own language, and in order to communicate clearly with the representatives, you need to be familiar with that language. See Box 6–1 for a listing of Insurance and Managed Care Terms.

APPLYING FOR PROVIDER STATUS

Identifying the HMO/insurance companies prevalent in your area is key. Make a list with the contact names, addresses, and telephone numbers that you want to target. There are directories available that may help you with this process. One directory is the *Nationwide Hospital Insurance Billing Directory*. Also, there is the Insurance Phone Book and Directory, published by the U.S. Directory Service. While you are compiling your list, you may want to ask other providers about the companies you are considering. You may learn that you do not want to deal with some of the companies on your list. You may gather your most valuable information by speaking with other nurse practitioners about their experiences with the specific companies. The American Academy of Nurse Practitioners is a valuable resource for learning more about nurse practitioner experience with managed care organizations. Your local, state, and national nurse practitioner meetings could be helpful when gathering this information.

Table 6-2	Medicaid State Agencies Web Addresses

Alabama
www.medicaid.state.al.us/

Alaska
www.hss.state.ak.us/

Arizona
www.ahcccs.state.az.us/

Arkansas
www.medicaid.state.ar.us/

California
www.medi-cal.ca.gov/

Colorado
www.state.co.us/

Connecticut
www.dss.state.ct.us/

Delaware
www.state.de.us/

District of Columbia
www.dchealth.com

Florida
www.fdhc.state.fl.us/

Georgia
www.state.ga.us/

Hawaii
www.state.hi.us/

Idaho
www2.state.id.us/

Illinois
www.state.il.us/

Indiana
www.dhs.state.ia.us/

Iowa
www.state.ia.us/

Kansas
www.srskansas.org

Kentucky
www.chs.state.ky.us/

Louisiana
www.dhh.state.la.us/

Maine
www.state.me.us/

Maryland
www.dhmh.state.md.us/

Massachusetts
www.state.ma.us/

Michigan
www.mdch.state.mi.us/

Minnesota
www.state.mn.us/

Mississippi
www.dom.state.ms.us/

Missouri
www.dss.state.mo.us/

Montana
www.dphhs.state.mt.us/

Nebraska
www.hhs.state.ne.us/

Nevada
www.state.nv.us/

New Hampshire
www.dhhs.state.nh.us/

New Jersey
www.state.nj.us/

New Mexico
www.state.nm.us/

New York
www.noah-health.org

North Carolina
www.dhhs.state.nc.us/

North Dakota
http://1notes.state.nd.us/

Ohio
www.state.oh.us/

Oklahoma
www.ohca.state.ok.us/

Oregon
www.omap.hr.state.or.us/

Pennsylvania
www.dpw.state.pa.us/

Rhode Island
www.dhs.state.ri.us/

South Dakota
www.state.sd.us/

Tennessee
www.state.tn.us/

Texas
www.hhsc.texas.gov

Utah
http://hlunix.hl.state.ut.us/

Vermont
www.dsw.state.vt.us/

Virginia
www.cns.state.va.us/

Washington
wws2.wa.gov

West Virginia
www.wvdhhr.org

Wisconsin
www.dhfs.state.wi.us/

Wyoming
http://wdhfs.state.wy.us/

Puerto Rico
www.valueoptions.com

Virgin Islands
www.gov.vi/health/

More information is available at
www.hcfa.gov/medicaid/medicaid.htm and
http://207.53.125/medicaid/states.htm.

Box 6–1
Insurance and Managed Care Terms

Capitation: A fee paid by a health maintenance organization (HMO) to a health-care provider, per patient, per month, for care of an HMO member. Capitated fees for primary care run on average between $5 and $35 per member per month, based on the patient's age and gender. Capitation may pay almost any health-care service, for example, primary care providers, specialty providers, ancillary services, hospital service, ambulance service, and prescriptions.

Carve Out: A health benefit—perhaps mental health care or dental care—that is removed from a larger benefits package and contracted separately to a specialized managed care organization.

Case Management: The coordination and integration of health services for patients with complex or extraordinarily costly medical problems, such as syndrome, spinal cord injury, and premature birth.

Closed Panel Model: A managed health plan that contracts with providers on an exclusive basis. The providers are not allowed to contract with other health plans.

Community Rating Method: an actuarial method for establishing a managed health plan's capitation rates.

Competitive Medical Plan: A managed health plan that qualifies for a Medicare risk contract without meeting some of the requirements needed to qualify as a health maintenance organization.

CPT Code: *Current Procedural Terminology*, a uniform coding system developed by the American Medical Association and adopted by third party payers for use in claim submission.

Deselection: The process by which a provider's participation in a managed health plan's network is terminated.

Disenrollment: The process by which a person's membership in a managed care plan is terminated. A member may disenroll voluntarily, perhaps to join another plan.

Exclusive Provider Organization: A preferred provider organization that requires its members to receive health care only from its provider network. Members are usually liable for out of plan medical care, except emergency care.

Fee-for-Service: Reimbursement for health-care services under a fee schedule. Fees are based on a complex variety of factors, including the number and type of services provided, the CPT and ICD-9 codes, the geographic area of service, and certain office and training expenses of the provider.

Group Model HMO: An HMO that contracts with a large practice to provide medical care to its members. The group may contract exclusively with and be partly owned by the HMO.

[Continued]

Health Maintenance Organization (HMO): A prepaid comprehensive system of health benefits that combines the financing and delivery of health services to subscribers. HMOs may pay providers on a fee-for-service or capitated bases. HMOs limit the providers they deal with to those only on their "panels."

Health Plan Employer Data and Information Set (HEDIS): A series of data elements that enable interested parties to calculate and compare numerous performance measures for HMOs. HEDIS is collected by the National Committee for Quality Assurance, a nonprofit organization that accredits HMOs that meet its quality of care standards. Performance measures involve such areas as quality, access, utilization, and finances.

ICD-9: *International Classification of Diseases*, 9th Revision. The classification of disease by medical diagnosis, codified into 6-digit numbers.

"Incident to" Services: The full term is "incident to a physician's professional service." A Medicare term, meaning services furnished as an "integral, although incidental, part of the physician's personal professional services in the course of diagnosis or treatment of an injury or illness." To qualify under this definition, the services of nonphysicians must be rendered under a physician's "direct personal supervision." Nonphysicians must be employees of a physician or a physician's group. Services must be furnished during a course of treatment in which a physician performs an initial service and subsequent services of a frequency that reflect the physician's active participation in the management of a course of treatment. Direct personal supervision in the office setting does not mean that the physician must be in the same room. However, a physician must be present in the office suite and immediately available to provide assistance and direction throughout the time a nurse practitioner is performing services.

Indemnity Insurer: An insurance company that pays for the medical care of the insured but does not deliver the health care.

Independent Practice Association (IPA)-model HMO: An HMO that contracts with numerous small independent group and solo practices through the intermediary that represents them. Providers maintain their individual practices and negotiate as a group with payers. The providers may be compensated on a capitated or fee-for-service basis.

Managed Behavioral Health Organization: A managed care organization that specializes in mental health care, which may include substance abuse services.

Managed Care: The systematic integration and coordination of the financing and delivery of health care. These activities are performed by health plans that try to provide their members with prepaid access to high-quality care at relatively low cost and usually are at least partly at risk for the cost of care. The health plans may rely on "gatekeepers" and prior authorization mechanisms to minimize unnecessary or inappropriate use of medical services.

Managed Care Organization (MCO): A preferred provider organization, provider-sponsored network, or any other health plan that integrates the financing and delivery or health care.

Managed Indemnity Plan: A health plan that reimburses providers on a fee-for-service basis but relies on preadmission certification, continued stay review, second surgical opinion, and other utilization management techniques.

Management Services Organization: An entity that performs claims processing, enrollment, marketing, and other management services for a health plan.

Medicaid: A federal program, administered by the states, for mother and children who qualify on the basis of poverty, and for adults who are disabled for the short term—1 year or less—and who qualify on the basis of poverty.

Medicaid Waiver: Permission to a state from the Health Care Finance Administration (HCFA) to administer Medicaid in ways that differ from the regulations, specifically to enroll patients covered by Medicaid in MCOs.

Medicare: A federal program, administered nationally by the HCFA and administered locally by Medicare carrier agencies. Medicare covers patients who are 65 years of age and older who have enrolled and pay premiums, and disabled individuals who qualify for Social Security disability payments and benefits.

National Committee on Quality Assurance (NCQA): A nonprofit, consumer-oriented group that rates managed care organizations on quality of care and sells the rating data to employers who purchase health plan services.

Network Model HMO: An HMO that contracts with several large single or multispecialty physician groups to provide medical care to its members.

Open Enrollment Period: A designated period, perhaps 1 to 2 months a year, during which a health plan's current members may switch health plans and nonmembers may apply for membership. State law may require a health plan to accept all applicants regardless of health status and prior coverage.

Open Panel Model: A managed health plan that contracts with providers who render care in their own offices. The provider may contract with other health plans.

Partial risk: The sharing of the financial risk associated with providing specific health services.

Physician Hospital Organization (PHO): An arrangement in which at least one hospital and one physician jointly provide health care services. The primary purpose of a PHO is to establish an organization that aligns physicians and hospitals to provide a full menu of health services.

Physician Organization (PO): POs are formed as joint ventures of primary care physicians for contracting with insurers and employers.

Preferred Provider Organization (PPO): A PPO is a contractual agreement between a panel of preferred providers and an insurance company, self-insured employer, third party administrator or manager, or managed care organization in order to provide services for fixed fees.

Reimbursement: Payment for services already delivered.

[Continued]

Risk Pool: An accounting fund that contains the withheld portions of providers' fees and capitation rates. Withheld amounts are at risk and are returned to the providers only if specific performance goals are met.

Stop Loss: The dollar threshold at which the provider's financial liability for additional care is greatly reduced or eliminated. The threshold may apply to each member individually or to all members combined. The threshold commonly is expressed on an annual basis. Once it is reached, the provider may be liable for only a small portion of all remaining costs.

Third Party Payer: An insurance company, HMO, or government agency that pays for medical services for a patient.

Usual and Customary: An insurance industry term for a charge that is (1) usual and customary, when compared with the charges made for similar services and supplies, and (2) made to persons having similar medical conditions in the county of the policy holder or such larger area than a county as needed to secure a representative cross section of fees.

Once you have your list together, call the *provider relations* department and inquire about the application process. The person you contact may be able to give you important information—make a friend, write down his or her name for future calls. Feel free to ask questions such as "Are there currently nurse practitioners on your provider panels? Has a nurse practitioner *ever* been admitted to your provider panel? What are the usual reasons for an applicant to be denied?" Take notes for future communications. Kindly request to have a provider application sent to you. Once you receive the application, fill it out clearly and completely. If you omit any information, you may receive the application back or you may receive a letter requesting the missing information. This will only slow the application process. Follow up with a telephone call if you haven't had a response within a couple of weeks. It may be tempting to apply before you even start your practice; however, the insurance companies may be looking at your track record. Many insurance companies require that you have been a licensed practitioner for at least 5 years as a prerequisite to becoming a provider. It may be best to wait to apply until after your practice is established. Managed care companies who are interested in contracting with you will investigate your education, license, certification, and other data on the application. They may or may not require a site visit. During the site visit, they will be assessing the cleanliness, safety, parking, staffing, signage, and so on of your site. After you have worked with them for a while, they may want to do a random chart review. They will also want to know about hospital admitting procedures as well as your system for contacting and communicating with your physician of protocol. They will also want to know how "after-hours" calls are handled. Do you have an answering service? Beeper? Cellular telephone?

Some practices really work at becoming accepted by as many plans as possible, or even just the choice plans. They prepare a promotional piece called a *practice analysis*, which basically demonstrates the value and uniqueness of the practice. Using real objective data, create a package that will convince the decision makers to select your practice to add to the provider panel. Some things to include in this package are the following:

- Curriculum vitae or resume
- Background information
- Copies of certification
- CME courses (show that the providers are growing and learning)
- Malpractice status (if cases are pending—explain)
- Hospital affiliations
- Letters from satisfied patients
- Description of office and staff
- Hours of operations (early, late, and weekend hours are a plus)
- Procedures done in office
- Routine screening schedule
- Payer profile (percentage of Medicare, Medicaid, self-pay, insured)
- Managed care experience
- Community service
- Copy of newsletter (if you produce one)
- Wellness handouts
- Statistics on cost effectiveness (e.g., fewer patients admitted to hospital, more patients get Pap smears, etc.)
- Website and e-mail communication with patients

If possible, document outcome data (e.g., number of referrals to specialists per 100 patients). Demonstrate patient satisfaction, survey patients on such topics as ease of making appointments, cleanliness of office, parking, and friendliness of staff. Show the advantages to them of contracting with your practice. There are consultants who can help you. It is best to hand deliver this package.

Once you are accepted and have been working with the managed care and insurance companies, try to evaluate the ease of working with each company. You may find it is not worth the time and effort to deal with certain companies. Evaluate the revenues versus the billing hassles.

CODING AND DOCUMENTATION

Coding is a special language within the health-care system. This is a language of codes and descriptions for health-care providers to use when billing insurance companies and other third-party payers for services provided. This is something you must know in a successful practice. Correct coding is required for payment. Many payments are delayed or rejected because of improper coding. There are basically two sets of coding that you need to be familiar with: *ICD-9-CM (International Classification of Diseases, Ninth Revision, Clinical Modification)* and *CPT (Current Procedural Terminology)*.

Many of the billing software programs have the CPT code built into the program library. Managed care authorizations will provide pre-approved CPT codes for services and procedures that are authorized.

ICD-9-CM codes were developed by the World Health Organization to describe patient complaints, conditions, diseases, injuries, and symptoms, as well as causes of morbidity and mortality. ICD-9-CM codes basically give a reason for the services provided. CPT codes were developed by the physicians at the American Medical Association to describe what providers do. CPT is the standard coding system for describing medical services and procedures. The CPT codes tell what services were provided. There are seminars and many books available to teach the basics of coding.

Your first step is to acquire the above-mentioned books (*ICD-9-CM*, Volumes 1 and 2 only—Volume 3 is for surgical procedures). Read through them and note what codes are applicable to your practice. If you know someone who is proficient in coding, ask him or her to teach you. There are professional coders and there is a certification test. If you are going to have a successful practice, you must have a good understanding of coding. Your coding must correlate with your patient notes. Your documentation must support the codes you have assigned. You must code to the highest level of specificity. You must code by the rules, not just by what the insurance will pay. You should buy new code books every year and have your coding staff attend seminars and read related articles and newsletters. Correct and accurate coding will maximize your revenues.

The Coding Institute in Naples, Florida, produces a monthly coding newsletter. More information on the *Nonphysician Practitioner Reimbursement Alert* is available at 1-800-508-2582.

THE REIMBURSEMENT PROCESS

If you are on the provider panels for HMO and insurance companies, you will have to comply with their specific billing procedures. Before patients are even scheduled for a visit, their insurance coverage must be verified. Some plans provide desktop software that allows you to check the patient's eligibility. Some may have the eligibility information available over the Internet or provide a terminal to swipe the patient's insurance card for verification. Photocopy the insurance card both front and back, and keep the copy in the patient's chart for future reference.

The front office staff should know (or have a list posted) of the insurance companies that require specific authorizations. The office manager should keep current with the changes with all of the plans. Keep all of the different plan information organized and handy for quick reference.

The nurse practitioner should take the responsibility of marking the superbill with the appropriate codes required for reimbursement. The documentation of the visit should include all of the same information related to the codes. For example, if a culture was obtained, it must be in the patient notes as well as on the superbill. Depending on the requirements of the insurance company, submit what they request (e.g., superbill, HCFA Form 1500, chart notes, treatment plan, summary). In the beginning, do the work yourself to learn the process. That way, you gain a strong foundation of knowledge in this potentially treacherous area. Once you have a good understanding of the billing process, you can work with your office staff to make sure that they are billing correctly. If you hire an office staff person who already has good experience and billing knowledge, then perhaps that person could teach you. Do not skip this very important step. By not following the coding and billing rules, you could not only be losing money with every patient, but you may also be charged with fraudulent billing.

Many different software packages are available for in-house billing at different levels of cost (e.g., *Medisoft, Medicserve, Medicomp*). You may want to learn about the differences in the programs. *Medisoft* is well known and used by many providers. Hiring the right person with good experience and references could greatly reduce your billing headaches and increase your reimbursement potential.

The following are tips for successful billing and reimbursement:

- Submit the insurance claim within 5 business days. It is optimal to submit all claims on the day of service. You cannot be paid until the claim form is submitted.
- Use superbills (keep them updated with current codes).
- Use the correct codes (extremely important).
- Follow each insurance company's rules for pre-authorization or pre-certification.
- Learn from your errors in billing and share the information with your billing staff.

If you have problems with slow payment, build a relationship with the claims representatives. Your requests for information and services will be documented, and these people can walk you through the process and help you identify the problems with your submissions—hopefully expediting your claims request.

BILLING SERVICES

Many practices use billing companies to assist in the billing process. Only if your practice has really grown quickly and things are out of hand would this be advisable. Billing companies charge an average of 10% of the total amount collected. Generally, billing from within your office is more cost effective. You may be contacted by different billing services that want to submit your claims to the insurance companies for you—for a fee, of course. Be careful. There are many stories of providers being taken advantage of by such companies. If you think about it, how can they know what level of service you provided, what procedures were done, what supplies were used, and what the diagnosis is unless you take the time to tell them? It may be tempting to let someone just take over an area of the business you don't really like dealing with; however, you may be setting yourself up for trouble.

If you decide to use this service, you must review all claims before they are submitted. Check all the codes; make sure you are both on the same track. Hire a company that allows the reimbursement checks to come directly to your mailing address. You can then Fax them the remittance forms for their records and invoice. It may be better to have one person in your office handle the billing. Be available to answer questions and help out. Remember, it is your reputation, license, and income that are on the line.

ETHICS AND BILLING

It may be tempting to "bend the rules" a little when billing. You may want to bill under your collaborating physician's name. You may want to exaggerate the extent of your actual patient care. Don't get greedy. Don't do it. You will live to regret it. As a nurse practitioner in independent practice, it is imperative that you follow the rules to the letter.

When dealing with managed care, nurse practitioners must be aware of potential ethical dilemmas or moral conflicts that may arise in a primary care setting. You want to provide quality patient care while working within a managed care environment that focuses on cost savings. Remember, you must provide complete, honest information to clients regarding choices for further diagnoses and treatment and regarding the constraints within the managed care system of their choice.

Medicare has increased substantially its investigations of health-care providers. You may not even know you are being investigated until it is too late. Don't put yourself in that position unnecessarily.

SUGGESTIONS AND TIPS FROM WOMEN'S HEALTH WATCH, INC.

■ Women's Health Watch, Inc., was designed and operated as a "cash practice." It was designed several years ago when most insurance providers had never heard of a nurse practitioner. It worked well for many years. However, in designing a practice for today and the future, it would certainly help maximize the revenue potential to include insurance and managed care companies.

- Credit cards proved their value time and time again. Not only for payment of office visits, but when doing collections it was wonderful to be able to get the credit card number and have the money owed deposited in our account within 48 hours. Also, for the cash-paying patient who also had a card, it was much easier to add on recommended testing and procedures on the same day.

PERSONAL ANECDOTES

1. I was very fortunate when hiring my office manager. She has been a close friend for years and is completely trustworthy. I had several local providers trying to steal her away from me. She has many years of insurance billing experience and is computer literate.

2. We kept a list of codes we used that were not on the superbill. The list was used as a quick reference and was also helpful when revising the superbill.

Resources

Abood, S, and Keepnews, D: Understanding payment for advanced practice nursing services. Medicare Reimbursement, Vol 1. American Nurses Publishing, Washington, DC, 2000.

American Medical Association, 515 N. State Street, Chicago, IL 60610: *www.ama-assn.org.*

American Medical Association: Physician's Current Procedural Terminology. AMA Books, Chicago, 2000.

American Medical Association: Assessing and Improving Billing and Collections (book and diskette). AMA Books, Chicago, 2000.

Buck, CJ, et al: Step-by-Step Medical Coding.WB Saunders, Philadelphia, 2000.

Buppert, C: Avoiding Medicare fraud, part 2. Nurse Practitioner 26:34–41, 2001.

Buppert, C: The Primary Care Provider's Guide to Compensation and Quality: How to Get Paid and Not Get Sued. Aspen, Gaithersburg, MD, 2000.

Davis, JB: Reimbursement Manual for the Medical Office: A Comprehensive Guide to Coding, Billing and Fee Management, 4th ed. Practice Management Information, Los Angeles, 2000.

Dunphy, LM, and Winland-Brown, JE: Primary Care: The Art and Science of Advanced Practice Nursing. FA Davis, Philadelphia, 2001.

Fordney, M: Insurance Handbook for the Medical Office. WB Saunders, Philadelphia, 1999.

Garofalo, WA, et al: Managed Care Contracting: A Practical Guide for Health Care Executives. Jossey Bass, San Francisco, 1999.

Insurance Phone Book and Directory, US Directory Service. Douglas Publications, New York, 2000.

Medicare Website: *www.hcfa.gov/medicare.*

Medicaid Website: *www.hcfa.gov/medicaid/medicaid.htm.*

Nationwide Hospital Insurance Billing Directory, Francis B. Kelly & Assoc., 123 Veteran Avenue, Los Angeles, CA 90024: 1-800-328-4144, *http://www.fbka.com.*

Nonphysician Practitioner Reimbursement Alert: 1-800-508-2582.

Office of Inspector General: *www.hhs.gov/oig.*

Swanson, K, and Lynch M: ICD-9 CM (Vols. 1–3). Practice Management Information, Los Angeles, 2000.

Credit Card Processing Companies

Bank of America: *www.bankamerica.com/merchant_services/home.html.*

Merchant Services/Nova Information Systems: *www.novainfo.com.*

PayNet Merchant Services: *www.visa-master.com.*

Billing Software

Medicserve: *www.medicserve.com.*

Medicomp: *www.erols.com.*

Medisoft: *www.medisoft.com.*

Coding Resources

Evaluation and Management Documentation Guidelines (2000): *www.hcfa.gov.*

United Communication Group: *www.ucg.com* 1-877-397-1496.

Newsletters & Seminars for Non-Physician Providers.

Nancy Maguire's Coding and Billing Expert Magazine.

Fraud & Abuse Answer Book (quarterly updates).

Nonphysician Practitioner Reimbursement Alert: 1-800-508-2582.

N O T E S

Chapter 7

Negligence and Liability: Defensive Medicine?

" I do the very best I know how—the very best I can; and I mean to keep on doing so until the end "

Abraham Lincoln

NEGLIGENCE

Your licensing board will respond to any report of nursing negligence. This includes gross negligence as well as reports of fraud, impairment, or criminal activity. Don't let this happen to you. Learn the laws of your state. Learn the Medicare and Medicaid rules. Then, follow them to the letter. Hopefully, this will help you practice safely within the law. Many states are now requiring some type of malpractice or liability insurance for nurse practitioners. Even if an insurance policy was not required for practice, it would be wise to protect yourself, your practice, and your assets with a good insurance policy. Hopefully, you will never have to notify the insurance company of an incident that could potentially develop into a lawsuit. But just think, wouldn't you feel a lot better having experienced professionals giving you guidance and protecting your license, practice, reputation, home, and savings?

RESEARCHING YOUR STATE LAWS

It is your responsibility as a licensed professional to research the laws of your state that pertain to your practice. You should research the laws, study the laws, and keep current copies on hand. In most states, when you receive your license, a copy of the state rules and statutes is included in the packet. If you do not have the laws in hand, you can usually access them through your licensing board's Website or via a telephone call to the board's office. If you have questions, contact your licensing board for clarification before it becomes an issue. See Chapter 5, Table 5–1, for licensing board contact information.

Now that you have the laws, have learned them, and are ready to practice, you need to become familiar with the definition of "standard of care" for your area of practice. There are many documents that define the "standard of care" for nurse practitioners. The traditional definition of "standard of care" includes "Acts performed that any other ordinary and prudent professional would have performed under the same or similar circumstances; the criterion by which professional performance is measured".[1]

Check with the American Academy of Nurse Practitioners, the American Nurses Association, and any specialty organizations for comprehensive definitions of "standard of care." Where is the line you don't cross in patient care? You could list out the skills or procedures you plan to perform with your practice—maybe follow the protocol example in Chapter 4. Know what you will do and, more importantly, what you will not do. Set your boundaries and stick to them. Discuss these rules with your collaborating physician—make sure he or she is comfortable with what you are planning to do with your independent practice. If you start to bend the rules, you will most likely find yourself in trouble. You are not doing yourself, your collaborating physician, or your patients any favors by stepping outside your comfort zone. Know when to refer—and do it.

FRAUD AND ABUSE

Fraud is simply defined as "deceit, trickery, and intentional deception." Abuse is simply defined as "to use wrongly, to mistreat, and to insult." None of these words sound like words you would like to hear associated with your name. In fact, you should be very careful to keep your reputation sparkling clean. When the terms "fraud" and "abuse" are heard regarding a medical practice, it usually has to do with improper billing to Medicaid, Medicare, and insurance companies.

Fraud committed by a nurse practitioner could include incorrect information on the nursing application to the state, falsifying medical records, or documenting something that has not been done—such as a patient visit. Examples of fraud include:

- Billing for goods/services not provided, or billing old items as new
- Incorrect reporting of diagnoses or procedures to receive higher payment
- Billing for covered services when non-covered services were provided
- Paying or receiving kickbacks, bribes, or rebates for patient referrals
- Routinely waiving deductibles or co-insurance
- Billing for phantom patient visits

- Billing for more hours than there are in a day
- Billing for unnecessary testing
- Inflating the bills for services provided
- Concealing ownership of related companies
- Falsifying credentials and double billing
- Fraudulent advertising

Medicare fraud has increased significantly over the past several years. To combat this increase, the U.S. Justice Department has increased its staff and investigative efforts in locating the source of fraud. You may have noticed advertisements by the Federal Bureau of Investigations (FBI) in the classified sections of nursing journals. The FBI is seeking information on provider fraud in the areas of hospitals, laboratories/clinics, nursing homes, home health care, medical transportation, and durable medical equipment. The FBI maintains regional fraud hotlines where calls are treated confidentially. You can get more information from their Website: *www.fbi.gov*. The FBI is not only looking for fraud in government-sponsored programs but also fraud in the private health insurance benefit programs. Physicians and nurse practitioners are not listed as part of the search for fraud, but I am sure they are looking for anyone associated with fraudulent practices. Your best defense is to have a staff that is devoted to billing correctly as well as to review every claim that goes out yourself. It will be you who will have to defend against charges, most likely not your employee.

It is your duty as a provider to be a "whistle blower" if you find gross fraudulent practices in your community. Before you make the call, make sure you have all the facts correct and as much evidence as possible. This action could backfire on you if you are wrong. If you do identify such practices, you have several options.

1. Call the Health and Human Services Inspector General's Hotline at 1-800-447-8477.
2. Write to Office of Inspector General, Department of Health and Human Services, 330 Independence Avenue SW, Washington, DC 20201.
3. Send an e-mail to *Htipds@os.dhhs.gov*.
4. Call Professionals Against Fraud for more information at 1-800-245-7154.

ILLEGAL KICKBACKS AND REBATES

Kickback—A giving back of part of money received as payment to referring provider.

Rebate—A return of part of a payment to the patient.

There are some fraudulent, devious schemes out there that make it financially beneficial for providers to refer or accept patients. Don't get greedy. A portion of the Social Security Act *provides criminal penalties for individuals or entities that knowingly and willfully offer, pay, solicit, or receive remuneration in order to induce business reimbursed under the Medicare or state health-care programs.* For a complete copy of the Medicare Anti-Kickback Statute, refer to *www.complianceland.com/aks/fedreg-7-29-91.html.* Heavy fines and imprisonment may be the end result if you decide to participate in illegal activity.

Even if you are not currently conducting any other business in the medical field besides running your practice, you will want to read through the section that explains "safe harbors." The 10 sections addressed under safe harbors include:

1. Investment interests
2. Space rental
3. Equipment rental
4. Personal services and management contracts
5. Sale of practice
6. Referral services
7. Warranties
8. Discounts
9. Employees
10. Group purchasing organizations

More information on safe harbors is available and can be easily found at: *www.complianceland.com/aks/fedreg-7-29-91.html.*

MALPRACTICE

Malpractice is defined as professional misconduct or improper conduct. Or, "the failure of a professional to exercise that degree of skill and learning commonly applied by the average prudent, reputable member of the profession".[1]

We have all heard too many stories of malpractice charges against local providers. In each case, try to identify where the provider first went wrong. Try to learn from their mistakes.

Use every chance you have to double check medications, chart notes, and all aspects of patient care. Do not be afraid to call your collaborating physician and refer patients if they need care that you cannot deliver safely. One thing you may want to research just for your own information is the statute of limitations in your state to file a malpractice claim. The statute of limitations is the time period in which a lawsuit can be filed.

Risk management is the practice of surveying a risk for potential sources of lawsuits and implementing actions designed to reduce injury.

If you are notified that you are being sued, your first call (after you calm down a little!) is to your liability insurance carrier. Have the chart handy, but DO NOT make any changes, do not add one word or remove any parts of it. It is probably the most tempting thing to do at the time, but that action can completely destroy your defense. Follow the instructions from your insurance carrier. Be very careful with whom you discuss the case. It may hurt your case if you speak too freely with the wrong people. Continue to practice. These matters can take years to resolve. Keep copies and notes of everything sent to your claims expert and your attorney. You will be assigned an attorney from your insurance company who will work with you to get the best end result possible. Share all of your records and recollections with this person. Be prepared to educate them not only on the role of the nurse practitioner, but also on the technical and medical aspects of the case. There will be a pretrial information gathering session. You will most likely be called to give a sworn deposition. Be very careful with your answers. Your attorney will be present and will have prepared you for most of the questions. Many cases are settled out of court to avoid the high costs of a court battle. Be very careful about agreeing to settle out of court. If you (or your insurance company) give the plaintiff money, it could appear as though you are admitting guilt. The settlement awards are recorded in the National Practitioner Data Bank. If you can avoid having such a finding on your record, do. Hopefully, this is an area you will never have to learn about first hand.

LIABILITY INSURANCE

Many states mandate that nurse practitioners carry their own liability (or malpractice) insurance. Selecting the correct policy is very important. There are basically two types of professional liability insurance plans: *claims-made* and *occurrence*.

A *claims-made* policy covers claims made against you only when the policy is in effect, meaning you must keep the policy active for as long as you are liable to ensure coverage for actions that occurred in the past. With the *occurrence policy*, you are covered for actions that occurred while the policy was in effect. "Tail coverage" is purchased with a claims-made policy to cover gaps in coverage that exist as a result of the nature of the claims-made policy. If you are canceling a claims-made policy, you may want to buy a few years of coverage to start immediately after the expiration date.

You must investigate the company from which you plan to purchase your malpractice insurance. If the company goes out of business, you are out of luck without coverage. *Best's Guide to Insurance Companies* is a book that rates insurance companies. Look up the company you are considering to purchase from to find their financial rating. This is definitely an area you should research—you want a quality company on your side if and when the time comes. See Box 7–1 for a listing of malpractice insurers for nurse practitioners.

Box 7–1

Malpractice Insurers for Nurse Practitioners

CM&F Group
151 William St.
New York, NY 10038
1-800-221-4904

Maginnis & Associates
Agency of Ohio
P.O. Box 543
Reynoldsburg, OH 43068-0543
1-614-866-3195

Nurse Protection Group
5 Airport Road
Lakewood, NJ 08701
1-800-545-4724
www.npg.com

Nurses Service Organization
4870 Street Road
Trevose, PA 19049
1-800-982-9491
www.nso.com

Seabury & Smith
Joan F. O'Sullivan, L.A.
75 Remittance Drive, Suite 1788
Chicago, IL 60675-1788
1-800-503-9230
www.seaburychicago.com

You must read through the policy to know exactly what your responsibilities are to the insurance company. Know what to do if there is an incident of concern—all the policies have different rules regarding when to contact the insurance company if you are concerned or know you are being sued. Know when you should contact them and what information you should have for them at that time. Know what your responsibilities are to the insurance company. More information about malpractice insurance is available at the NP Central Website: *www.nurse.net.*

MINIMIZING MALPRACTICE RISKS

As a rule, most patients are not able to judge the quality of a health-care provider's service. However, they can and will judge a practitioner and their staff on their interpersonal skills. And, as silly as this may sound, the interpersonal skills/relationship usually determines whether a patient will sue or not.

> *It will come as no surprise that the majority of patients who have sued their physicians have stated: I would never have sued my doctor if he/she would only have:*
>
> ■ *Been honest*
> ■ *Said they were sorry*
> ■ *Listened to me*
> ■ *Acted like they cared*[2]

Communication is key to a successful practice. Introduce yourself to your new patients and wear a nametag. Don't use medical terms they won't understand. Never guarantee an outcome or criticize another provider. Before a procedure, take the extra time to explain what the patient should expect, what to do to prepare, and answer all questions to the best of your knowledge. Do not interrupt the patient. Do not talk down to the patient. Slow down—don't rush through explanations, and truly listen to your patient. Return all telephone calls as soon as possible.

Learn how to identify "potential" problem patients before they become "real" problem patients! This is the patient who never seems to be satisfied. When you have a difficult patient, be sure to cover yourself. You may want to have staff members in the room with you when seeing the patient, document every interaction carefully, have the staff record all interactions clearly in the chart, recommend a second opinion, do whatever you can to get this patient to understand that you are working with them to find answers. Problem patients may be resentful, angry, and dissatisfied. Document their statements and never admit to any wrongdoing. Conduct a through assessment—both emotional and physical—and document educational methods used. Demonstrate in your documentation that you took the complaint seriously and did everything you could for the patient.

Educational materials given to the patient may help your case more than you know. Not only are they time savers but they may also be lifesavers. The educational material may contain information regarding the diagnosis, procedure, and medications. This may take away the claim that the patient was never told certain things. Document the exact handout given to the patient; it may be important someday. Keep copies of all handouts with the dates they were used at your practice, even after they have been retired.

An obvious indicator of a potential lawsuit would be an unexpected outcome or complications during the treatment of your patient. Or, perhaps, the first sign of a problem could be that an attorney contacts you for copies of a patient record. Remember, most malpractice lawsuits never go to trial. And, just because someone claims you did something wrong doesn't mean that you did something wrong!

NATIONAL PRACTITIONER DATA BANK

More than 10 years ago, the Department of Health and Human Services (HHS) instituted the National Practitioner Data Bank (NPDB). The NPDB is an information clearinghouse that collects and releases information related to the professional competence and conduct of physicians, nurse practitioners, dentists, and some other health-care practitioners. The NPDB contains information on malpractice payments, adverse licensure actions, certain negative professional review actions, and reports of Medicare and Medicaid sanctions. Hospitals, managed care organizations, and insurance companies are among the entities that can request reports from the NPDB. If you (or your insurance company) pay a malpractice settlement, you must report it to the NPDB. Failure to report the payment may result in a $10,000 fine. You may request a report on yourself. The information is available at *www.npdb.com* or 1-800-767-6732.

FINAL THOUGHTS ON MALPRACTICE

Malpractice is one of the "dirtiest" words known to health-care providers. We did not go into this line of work to inflict harm or cause damage to human beings. However, it is not realistic to ignore the fact that too many providers are sued. "Realistically it's not necessary to worry about the threat of malpractice on a day-to-day basis. The best advice is to keep current in your field, document well, and if you do not know, ask or consult".[3]

OTHER INSURANCE TO CONSIDER: WHAT IF THE UNEXPECTED HAPPENS?

You do not want to waste your hard-earned money by buying unnecessary insurance policies. However, everyone's situation is different. If you are the head of the household and everyone depends on your income to live, you may want to consider some other types of insurance. As with malpractice insurance, you hope you never have to call upon the insurance company for payment, but then again, if something bad happened to you, wouldn't you feel a lot better having money to pay your mortgage and buy groceries?

The key to getting the best and most insurance coverage for your money is having good advisors who will look at your total package. Instead of buying several different policies from several different insurance agents, try to coordinate your efforts. Many of the policies may overlap and you may find yourself overpaying for coverage of the same items on different policies. You should enlist the services of a certified financial planner or a good insurance broker to oversee your entire insurance coverage.

Disability Insurance

Can you imagine trying to live without a paycheck for an extended amount of time, possibly forever? With statistics showing that more than 1 in 10 people age 25 to 64 suffers a disability, we should be buying disability insurance to protect our assets, our families, and ourselves. Disability insurance may seem a bit expensive, but the premiums average 1 to 3 percent of your income. If you decide to purchase disability insurance, be sure to go through a reputable insurance agent and use a reputable insurance company.

Even though many people may have purchased and wonder whether they have enough life insurance, they should really be thinking about disability insurance. Disability is as important, if not more important, than life insurance. The basic rule is this: If you are working and you need your income to live, then you need disability insurance. Don't be fooled that Social Security will protect you if you are disabled—more than 80 percent of the applicants for Social Security are rejected the first time they apply. Social Security has very stringent qualifying requirements for disability claims, and the amount paid is usually meager.

There are many different types of disability policies. By working with your insurance broker, you should be able to find an appropriate policy for you in regard to:

- The amount of monthly benefit (e.g., fixed amount, cost of living raises)
- The definition of disability ("own occupation" or "any occupation")
- The waiting period for the policy to go into effect after the disability occurs (1 week to 2 years; most common is 60 to 90 days.)
- The benefit period—how long you will receive monthly benefits (6 months to life)
- The insurance policy premium amounts and schedule (monthly, quarterly, annually)
- The qualifying data—income, occupation, and medical and mental health history

Over the years, it has become more and more difficult to obtain disability insurance. Unfortunately, this is an area where fraud has become prevalent. If you choose to purchase disability insurance, try to get:

- The highest monthly benefits for which you can qualify.
- "Own occupation" coverage for life so you aren't forced into working in a new line of work. You may want to try to attach your management protocol that specifically outlines your daily work activities.

▪ The longest waiting period you can afford. A policy with a 6-month waiting period is much less expensive than a 2-week waiting period.

▪ Coverage for the longest period possible—age 65 or life.

Hopefully, you will never have to request benefits for this type of policy, but what if...? Just think of the peace of mind you could experience if you have prepared yourself with disability insurance and you are facing living with a disability.

Business Owners' Insurance

There are two different forms of property insurance for buildings and contents owned by the company: standard and special. These provide comprehensive coverage. Business interruption insurance covers the loss of income resulting from a fire or other catastrophe that disrupts the operation of the business. It can also include the extra expense of operating out of a temporary location.

Business Umbrella Policy

This insurance covers things that are not protected in your traditional business owners insurance policy. These policies usually have higher limits than the business owners insurance policies and can help fill in the gaps for areas that are not covered in your other policies.

Personal Umbrella Policy

This is an insurance contract designed to accomplish two goals. (1) The liability protection is increased for current homeowners and auto insurance policies. (2) It is also designed to fill in the gaps with other liability insurance policies because many activities are not covered under traditional policies.

The personal umbrella policy is really designed to give you extra protection against lawsuits that are not covered with your other insurance policies. This can be very important coverage if someone is in a motor vehicle accident or boating accident, or is injured in your home. It is relatively inexpensive and is easier to obtain than the disability insurance policies.

Personal umbrella policies usually are available with $1 to $5 million liability limits. Similar to other insurance policies, many variables determine premium payment amounts. Remember, the more you own, the more you have to protect. And, no matter how careful you are, sometimes accidents occur that are not covered with your everyday insurance policies.

Rental Insurance

If you rent your office space, you are responsible for loss or damage to your belongings and for damages resulting from injuries inside your door. As a rule, your landlord is not responsible for such disagreeable situations. Renter's insurance covers most property losses and typically pays legal fees as well as any adverse settlement. If you keep computers, medical equipment, cash, or art objects worth more than $5,000 in your office, consider paying a little extra for "floater" coverage of such high-ticket items.

Disaster Insurance

There are many things beyond your control when it comes to natural disasters. However, there are a few things you can do in advance to protect yourself and your practice. Besides securing your property and keeping everything in good repair, there are additional types of insurance to cover you during these events. Disaster insurance may be available to you for earthquakes, fires, floods, hurricanes, and tornadoes. This is an area where you must evaluate and decide whether the cost of the premium is worth the available coverage. These policies also vary with your location in the United States and the potential natural disasters that are common in your location. Make sure you are not paying for this coverage in more than one of your policies.

Health Insurance

Being a health-care provider, you must have an idea of what type of insurance you would like for you and your family. When developing your employee benefit package, you may need to purchase insurance for your employees. There are essentially two types of health insurance: (1) fee for service and (2) managed care. A good insurance agent will be able to provide you all of the required information and rates that will help you decide what policy is right for you, your family, and your employees.

Life Insurance

The main goal of obtaining life insurance traditionally has been to protect your family from financial ruin in the event of your death. There are two basic life insurance policies available: term and permanent.

Term life insurance is good for some people because it usually is initially low cost and the most affordable option. The premiums usually increase during your later years and people tend to drop the coverage just when they need it the most. Permanent life insurance is a good long-term coverage with stable premiums and has a cash value while you are living.

Another area to consider is life insurance for your spouse or significant other. Think of the potential economic devastation that would occur if you lost that person's income. Even if he or she doesn't bring in a paycheck, think of what it may cost you to replace their daily duties—nanny, housekeeper, cook, driver, and so on. You may not like to think about losing people you love, but these things should be thought out so you are better prepared to deal with these issues.

Summary

Take the time to review all of your policies and their coverage with your certified financial planner or your insurance broker. It is good for you to take the time to learn what your policies actually cover in case you ever need them.

SUGGESTIONS AND TIPS FROM WOMEN'S HEALTH WATCH, INC.

- Purchase your liability insurance from a large company that covers other nurse practitioners. You may want to submit a copy of your protocol so they know what you are doing within your practice. Keep the front sheet of the policy handy. If you are working elsewhere, they may require a copy of the face sheet.

- Many policies allow you to purchase coverage for your business and your office staff. It may be wise to do so. You want the best coverage you can get, but you do not want to have more insurance payments due than patient payments coming in!

PERSONAL ANECDOTES

1. Fortunately, I don't have any personal experience with malpractice (knock on wood!). However, after practicing in "Litigious South Florida," I do have plenty of experience in wondering and worrying about malpractice lawsuits. I felt I needed to look at every patient as a potential lawsuit—to communicate clearly, answer all questions, provide the best care possible, show my concern, and document clearly and thoroughly.

2. Hopefully, you will not have to deal with a lawsuit. If you do, take it one day at a time—hopefully, the case will fall apart before it develops into a real case.

Resources

American Academy of Nurse Practitioners: *www.aanp.org.*
American Nurses Association: 1-800-274-4ANA.
Best's Guide to Insurance Companies [online]. AM. Best Company, *www.ambest.com.*
Carroll, R: Risk Management Handbook, 2nd ed. American Hospital Publishing, Chicago, 1990.
Certified Financial Planners Directory: *www.fpanet.org/plannersearch/index.cfm.*

Department of Health and Human Services Hot Tips: *Htipds@os.dhhs.gov.*
Federal Bureau of Investigations: *www.fbi.gov.*
HHS Inspector General's Hotline: 1-800-447-8477.
Insurance Broker—B&B Coverage LTD: *www.bbcoverage.com* or 516-872-2300.
Katz, S, and Goldberg, D: 2003. Personal interview regarding insurance policies. Ft. Lauderdale, Florida.
Malpractice Insurance Information, NP Central Website: *www.nurse.net.*
Medicare Anti-Kickback Statute: *www.complianceland.com/aks/fedreg-7-29-91.html.*
Morrison, CA: Tracking through data banks. Advances for Nurse Practitioners 2:25, 2001.
Morrison, CA: Become more legally aware. Advances for Nurse Practitioners 11:32, 2000.
National Practitioner Data Bank: *www.npdb.com* or 1-800-767-6732.
Office of Inspector General, Department of Health and Human Services, 330 Independence Avenue SW, Washington, DC 20201.
Rice, B: It's a physician's duty to expose fraud if he suspects it. Medical Economics [online, 1999]:
http://www.pdr.net/memag/public.htm?path=docs/092099/article4.html.
Shaw, M: Nurses Legal Handbook, 3rd ed. Springhouse Corp, Springhouse, PA, 1996.

References

1. Buppert, C: Nurse Practitioner's Business Practice and Legal Guide. Aspen, Gaithersburg, MD, 1999.
2. Allen, D: It's the little things you do that prevent malpractice litigation. Florida Medical Business Jan. 26, 1999, p 13.
3. Miller, SK: Are NPs overly concerned about malpractice? Patient Care for the Nurse Practitioner 7:74, 2000.

NOTES

Chapter 8

Hospital Privileges: Do I Really Need Them?

" Nothing happens unless first a dream "

Carl Sandburg

Hospital privileges can be very important to the nurse practitioner's ability to practice fully. Each hospital has its own process of screening applicants to ensure that it has qualified, competent providers on staff. Many factors can influence the credentialing committee or hospital board. Researching the information that will help you with a successful application is time well spent.

WHAT ARE "HOSPITAL PRIVILEGES?"

Each hospital has its own governing rules for providers who practice under their roof. The different privilege levels are defined by the medical staff governing body and may be *full, limited, associate, affiliate, temporary, consultant,* or any other term the governing body decides upon. It is important for you to know the levels of privileges available for nurse practitioners and what level of privilege you think is needed for your practice *before* you apply. The levels of practice range from "full" privileges, wherein the practitioner has the ability to admit, discharge, and order medications and treatments just like their physician colleagues, to clinical "affiliate" privileges, which in many hospitals is the designation used for any nonphysician provider. This level of privilege often restricts the practitioner's scope of practice to one of a physician extender. There is usually a comprehensive application process to complete before one is granted hospital privileges.

EVALUATING YOUR NEED FOR HOSPITAL PRIVILEGES

Some types of practices can function without hospital privileges and not be affected adversely. A few questions to ask yourself, to help you decide whether you need hospital privileges include:

- What type of practice do you plan on opening?
- How will you handle patients who need to be admitted?
- Will you apply to become a primary care provider with insurance companies?
- Will the insurance companies require hospital privileges?
- How are the relations between the local doctors and the local nurse practitioners?
- Are any nurse practitioners currently admitting at this hospital?
- Are applications for privileges from nurse practitioners being accepted at your local hospital?

THE APPLICATION PROCESS

The application process can be a nerve-racking and time-consuming process that should not be taken lightly. If you casually submit an incomplete or inaccurate application and you are denied privileges, that denial of privileges will stay on your record for the rest of your career. You want to know that you have a good chance of receiving your requested privileges *before* you submit your application. Contact the medical staff office of the hospital to which you are applying for privileges to learn whether there are already nurse practitioners with privileges at the hospital. Inquire about the application process, how to obtain an application, and how long it takes before a decision is made regarding your application once it has been submitted.

Request a copy of the by-laws of the professional staff from the hospital. The by-laws outline the application process and the medical staff rules in more detail. If there are already nurse practitioners on staff, the process may be as simple as filling out one sheet of questions regarding what functions you would like to perform in the hospital and having your "sponsoring physician" sign the form. This type of simple application may require that the sponsoring physician countersign all chart entries. See Figure 8–1 for a sample of this type of application. Be certain you know what your level of practice privileges allow you to do.

Most hospitals require a more extensive application, requiring information about your education, licensure, certifications, training, hospital staff history,

| **Figure 8–1** | **Sample Application for Privileges for Nurse Practitioners** |

Name _____

Name of facility where you desire privileges: _____

INSTRUCTIONS: The nurse practitioner should check those privileges desired. The nurse practitioner will be under the supervision of a sponsoring physician.

CHECK FUNCTIONS REQUESTED:	**REQUESTED**	**APPROVED**
1. Interview patient for medical history and examine patient.	☐	☐
2. Dictate and/or write history and physical (to be countersigned by physician within 24 hours).	☐	☐
3. Initiate, select, and modify selected medications and/or therapies for management of disease/illness (to be countersigned by physician within 24 hours).	☐	☐
4. Dictate and/or write progress notes (to be countersigned by physician within 24 hours).	☐	☐
5. Dictate and/or write discharge summaries (to be countersigned by physician within 24 hours).	☐	☐
6. Provide instruction on nutrition, physical exercise, therapy, and other aspects of care (to be countersigned by physician within 24 hours).	☐	☐
7. Other _____	☐	☐
8. Other _____	☐	☐

_____   _____

Signature of Applicant   Date

_____   _____

Signature of Sponsoring Physician   Date

_____   _____

Signature of Chief of Staff   Date peer references, malpractice insurance information, personal health, and other professional information. Supporting documents may be requested, including proof of malpractice insurance, proof of licensure and certification, curriculum vitae, photograph, letters of recommendation, and certified copies of diplomas. There may be an application fee and possibly an annual fee for hospital privileges.

Answer all questions on the application clearly and completely. Try to make a contact or friend in the medical staff office who you can call to check on the progress of your application. After you have completed the form, find out who will be reviewing the application (who is on the credentialing committee) and when it will be reviewed.

DENIAL OF PRIVILEGES

If you are denied privileges, don't take this as your final answer. Ask questions and find out what you need to do to be granted privileges. Be persistent, but do not be rude. Keep trying until you succeed. Some hospitals have a designated period of time before you can reapply. Make sure you know all the rules and regulations. Lawsuits have been filed by health-care providers who were denied hospital privileges. Of course, you would want to exhaust all other options before taking on the expense and emotion of a legal battle.

SUGGESTIONS AND TIPS FROM WOMEN'S HEALTH WATCH, INC.

- When designing Women's Health Watch, I made a conscious decision to create a practice that did not include hospital care. The business was designed and operated basically as "office gynecology." When a patient required hospitalization, she was referred to a local physician for care.

- One of the benefits of not having hospital privileges was that it removed a potential board of physicians looking into my practice. I thought that they could possibly have an adverse impact on my practice by questioning or dictating my patient care.

PERSONAL ANECDOTES

1. Even though I didn't need (or want) hospital privileges, I found myself involved in the application process in an indirect way. I was serving as a clinical instructor at some of the local nurse practitioner programs for several years. Many of the students who graduated used my name as a

reference on their application for hospital privileges. Because I had worked with them in the clinical area, I was able to give strong, convincing recommendations. You may want to call upon past instructors for recommendations.

2. Having a little paranoia about being the only nurse practitioner in independent practice in the area, it felt good that the local physicians did not have any control over my practice. The only physician I had to answer to was my collaborating physician, and he was such a fan of nurse practitioners that I didn't need to worry.

Resources

Bischel, MD: The Credentialing and Privileges Manual. Apollo Managed Care Consultants, Santa Barbara, 1999.

Levin, LM: Medical Staff Privileges: A Practical Guide to Obtaining and Keeping Hospital Staff Privileges. Practice Management Information Corporation, Los Angeles, 1996.

Pollard, MJ, and Wigal, GJ: Hospital Staff Privileges: What Every Hospital, Administrator, Physician, Health Care Provider and Lawyer Needs to Know. Health Administration Press, Chicago, 1995.

Rozovsky, FA, et al: Medical Staff Credentialing: A Practical Guide. American Hospital Publishing, Chicago, 1993.

Tomes, J: Medical Staff Privileges and Peer Review. Probus Publishing, Chicago, 1994.

N O T E S

Chapter 9

Prescriptive Privileges: What Do I Need to Do with Prescriptions?

" The price of power is responsibility for the public good "

Winthrop W. Aldrich

It is your duty as a licensed professional to know the laws of the state in which you practice. As you know, prescriptive laws vary from state to state. Some nurse practitioners have full privileges, meaning they can write prescriptions for all medications, whereas some states have stringent rules and regulations limiting the nurse practitioner's prescriptive privileges.

REGULATIONS

To locate the prescriptive regulations for the state in which you practice, you may contact the licensing board. Usually, you receive a copy of the laws relating to your practice when you receive your license. The January issue of *The Nurse Practitioner Journal* includes an annual update of how each state stands on legislative issues affecting advanced nursing practice. This update is comprehensive, including sections on legal authority, reimbursement, and prescriptive authority. This is an excellent resource. The Drug Enforcement Administration (DEA) has information on "mid-level practitioners authorization by state" (prescriptive privileges) available at their Website: *www. deadiversion.usdoj.gov/drugreg/practitioners/index.html.*

PRESCRIBING PRACTICES

The information printed and written on prescription pads must comply with the state statutes and rules relating to nurse practitioner practice. Refer to your licensing board or the materials you received with your license. The basic information that must be included on all prescriptions includes:

- Name, title, address, and phone number of the nurse practitioner who is prescribing
- Full name and address of the patient
- Date of issuance of the prescription
- The full name of the drug, dosage, route, quantity, and clear directions for its use; avoid "p.r.n" and "as directed"
- Number of refills authorized
- Signature of the prescriber with appropriate degree and certification initials

Other information that may be required by the state or you may choose to include:

- DEA number of the prescriber
- Full name and academic degree of the collaborating or supervising physician
- Prescriber's license number
- Age or date of birth of the patient
- "Substitution permissible," "do not substitute," "medically necessary" with check off boxes

Prescription pads can be printed with single tear off sheets, or with carbonless copies. Having a true copy of the prescription written can be very helpful when questions arise. Telephone calls from the patient or pharmacist can be answered easily and quickly by referring to the copy. Legally, wouldn't it be ideal to have a copy of the prescription in the chart? You may be eligible to receive complimentary printed prescription pads from pharmaceutical companies; if you want them, ask your local representative. You may also qualify to receive free prescription pads from Triple I Prescription Pads (1-800-969-7237).

When calling in prescriptions to the pharmacy, be sure to give all the required information. Speak slowly and clearly in a pleasant voice. Be sure to leave the office telephone number so the pharmacist can call with any questions.

DRUG ENFORCEMENT ADMINISTRATION

The DEA registers health-care providers who prescribe controlled dangerous substances. The DEA refers to nurse practitioners as "mid-level practitioners." Nurse practitioners who are permitted by their state laws to prescribe controlled substances must register with the DEA and will receive a DEA number once their application is approved. You must also have a practice site and no felony record. The DEA now offers online registration for nurse practitioners at *www.DEAdiversions.usdoj.gov*. Applications for registration may be obtained from any DEA office with diversion staff. You can find the office closest to you and learn more about the DEA registration process by calling 1-800-882-9539 or at their Website: *www.deadiversion.usdoh.gov/drugreg/process/htm*. The processing and issuing of a DEA registration usually takes 6 to 8 weeks when the application is filled out completely and correctly. The DEA has compiled the *Mid-Level Practitioner's Manual*, which can be accessed at *www.deadiversion.usdoj.gov/pubsd/manualsd/index.html*. Through this same Website, you can access the prescriptive laws for each state regarding nurse practitioners.

DISPENSING

The state in which you practice may have specific rules and regulations regarding the dispensing of pharmaceuticals from your office. The state may require a special "dispensing license." Recently, there has been an increase in the number of health-care providers who dispense (sell) the medications they prescribe for their patients from their office. This is not only a way to increase office revenues, but it is also provides convenience and savings for patients. Ten to twenty percent of doctors are dispensing medications and the percentage is increasing.

Companies such as Physicians Total Care (*www.physianstotalcare.com*) offer programs that electronically connect medical offices to HMO pharmacy benefit managers for immediate claims adjudication and confirmation of reimbursement. The program also fully automates the dispensing process and inventory control. Several companies are providing medications that are prepackaged and sealed in counts commonly dispensed. Computer systems in some dispensing machines print labels at the time of dispensing. Pyxis (*www.pyxis.com*), Darby Drug Company (*www.darbydrug.com*), Florida Infusion (*www.floridainfusion.com*), and Kraft Pharmaceuticals (1-800-887-5155) are companies that also provide automated medication dispensing systems and medications.

ELECTRONIC PRESCRIBING SYSTEMS

The number of states that allow electronically transmitted prescriptions (also referred to as electronic prescribing systems) has been rising in the past several years. The benefits to the patient and the provider are substantial. It is speculated that the number of medication errors will be greatly reduced with electronically transmitted prescriptions. These prescriptions may be transmitted to local pharmacies or online pharmacies. To send electronically transmitted prescriptions, you must obtain a *personal digital assistant (PDA)*, computer, modem, software, printer with infrared or radio-transmission receiver, internet link, or designated connection. Some companies that provide the equipment and service are Allscripts (*www.allscripts.com*), PocketScript (*www.pocketscript.com*), and iScribe (*www.iscribe.com*).[1] Several companies are developing and supplying the electronic units.

ONLINE PHARMACIES

Online pharmacies hold appeal to many patients. Some of the benefits of online pharmacies for the patient include:

- Lower medication prices
- Round-the-clock ordering capabilities
- No long wait standing at the pharmacy
- Delivery to doorstep
- Automatic e-mail reminders for refills
- Increased autonomy for the patient (more medication information on Websites)

Downsides of using an online pharmacy include:

- Some may not be equipped to receive prescriptions electronically.
- Out-of-state pharmacies may have a problem filling prescriptions because of state laws.
- There may be a delay in receiving prescriptions because of mail delivery.
- More telephone calls and questions are directed to the provider.

BE THE PATIENT'S ADVOCATE

Pharmaceutical representatives are eager to teach you everything there is to know about the medications produced by the company they represent. They will also supply you with samples of medications, patient educational literature, promotional products (e.g., pens, note pads, magnets). They may also sponsor local and national meetings to help educate prescribers on the benefits of their products. The medication samples given to you to give to patients can help your patients reduce their pharmacy bill. You must supply the patient with literature on the medication, even when you are giving them samples. There have been malpractice lawsuits in the past when a patient was given sample medication and had a severe adverse reaction. The provider had not given the patient the medication literature with the sample. The provider lost the case. Write out the medication instructions clearly for the patient.

Learn the costs of the medications you prescribe. Some patients won't be able to afford the medication prescribed and won't get the prescription filled. It is good to be able to give them an idea of what the prescription will cost them if they don't have insurance. Talk with them about whether they will be able to find a way to get the prescription filled. Find less costly alternative medications and supplement the prescription with samples when you can.

Many of the large pharmaceutical companies have programs to help low income patients receive their medication free. To find out about the programs available, contact the pharmaceutical company that supplies the needed medication and ask to be connected with the "patient assistance program." Request a list of covered medications and enrollment applications. You will also find a list of patient assistance programs along with more information at the Website of the Pharmaceutical Research and Manufacturers of America (*www.phrma.org/patients*). Another program, RxAssist, is an online tool created to assist health-care providers in locating sources of free pharmaceuticals for uninsured patients (*www.rxassist.org*).

PRESCRIPTION FRAUD

As you know, prescription drug abuse (especially controlled substances) is a serious social and health problem in the United States. As a health-care professional, you have responsibilities to help correct and prevent further abuses. Legally and ethically, it is your responsibility to uphold the law and help protect society from drug abuse. If you are prescribing controlled substances, you have a professional responsibility to prescribe appropriately, guarding against abuse, while ensuring that your patients get the medications they need. Personally, you have the responsibility to protect your practice and license from becoming an easy target for fraud. You must do everything you can to prevent prescription fraud and abuse.

Keep all of your prescription pads in a safe place, out of the sight and reach of patients. Learn to recognize the common characteristics of the drug abuser. More information on identifying the drug abuser is available at *www.deadiversion.usdoj.gov/pubs/brochures/drugabuser.htm*.

Usually, prescription fraud involves someone changing the information on a legitimate prescription or someone trying to write his or her own prescriptions. A person may try to call in a prescription to the pharmacy or even steal your prescription pad. With computers, such people may actually generate fake prescriptions that look like the ones you have in your office. To safeguard your practice, keep prescription pads in a safe place and develop a healthy suspicion of anyone trying to elicit your personal data (e.g., license number, DEA number, signature, letterhead).

Many providers require patients to sign a written agreement regarding narcotics prescribed for pain. The agreement documents what is required by the patient and can prevent misunderstandings (Fig. 9–1).

SUGGESTIONS AND TIPS FROM WOMEN'S HEALTH WATCH, INC.

- To handle the requirement of providing patients written material on all medications prescribed and sampled, we devised a great filing system. We kept it close to the sample cupboard and worked at complying with the laws. The pharmaceutical representatives may be able to provide the written material appropriate for the patient. If not, you can easily create them and reproduce them on the copy machine.

- To make alterations of the prescriptions more difficult, spell out the number of pills and the number of refills. You want to do everything you can to prevent fraud.

- Never use prescription pads as note pads or for memos. Treat your prescription pad like you treat your checkbook. Keep it safe and tucked away.

PERSONAL ANECDOTES

1. During my first week of working as a nurse practitioner, a patient manipulated me into writing a prescription for a narcotic cough syrup. After she left, I went into a major panic. In Florida, we were not allowed to write prescriptions for controlled substances. I called my physician of protocol and confessed what I had done. He said I should relax and that he would authorize the prescription, but I was to learn from this experience. I did. I became very aware of patients requesting specific medications and I came up with the perfect line: "I cannot write that prescription, it is against the law." They would usually give up when I mentioned the law. I would offer them a referral to a physician to help ease the rejection.

2. I received an interesting call from a nurse practitioner in Miami who wanted my advice. She had been contacted by the DEA regarding some prescriptions she had written for controlled substances. She asked what she should do. I told her she might want to hire an attorney because she had broken the law. She said she had been practicing as a nurse practitioner and writing prescriptions for controlled substances in Florida for more than 12 years! She said she didn't know she wasn't supposed to be writing for controlled substances! What is it they say about ignorance?

Figure 9–1	Controlled Substance Agreement

The purpose of this agreement is to prevent misunderstandings about certain medicines you will be taking prescribed by your nurse practitioner. This is to help both you and your nurse practitioner comply with the laws regarding controlled substances.

- I understand that this agreement is essential to the trust and confidence necessary in a nurse practitioner/patient relationship and that my nurse practitioner undertakes to treat me on this agreement.

- I understand that if I break this agreement, my nurse practitioner will stop prescribing these medications.

- In this case, my nurse practitioner will taper off the medicine over a period of several days, as necessary, to avoid withdrawal symptoms. Also, a drug dependence treatment program may be recommended.

- I will communicate fully with my nurse practitioner in describing the severity of my pain, how the pain affects my daily life, and how well the medicine is helping me.

- I will not attempt to buy or use any illegal controlled substances, such as marijuana or cocaine.

- I will not share, trade, or sell my pain medication with anyone.

- I will not attempt to obtain any controlled medicines, including pain medications, controlled stimulants, or antianxiety medicines from any other nurse practitioner or physician.

- I will keep my medication in a safe place. Lost or stolen medications will not be replaced.

- I agree that refills for my prescriptions for the controlled substances will be made only during scheduled appointments or during regular office hours. No refills will be available during evenings or on weekends.

- I authorize my nurse practitioner and my pharmacy to cooperate fully with any city, state, or federal law enforcement agency, including this state Board of Pharmacy, in the investigation of any possible misuse, sale, or other diversion of my medication. I authorize my nurse practitioner to provide a copy of this agreement to my pharmacy. I agree to waive any applicable privilege or right of privacy or confidentiality with respect to these authorizations.

- I agree that I will submit to a blood or urine test if requested by my nurse practitioner to determine my compliance with my medication program.

- I agree that I will use my medicine at a rate no greater than prescribed rate and that use of my medicine at a greater rate will result in my being without medication for a period of time.

- I will bring all unused pain medication to every office visit.

- I agree to follow these guidelines that have been fully explained to me. All of my questions and concerns regarding treatment have been adequately answered. A copy of this document has been given to me.

Date:_____

Patient signature_____

Nurse practitioner signature_____

Witness_____

Adapted from *Opioid Therapy Documentation Kit by Elizabeth J. Narcessian, MD, for Purdue Pharma, L.P.*

Resources

Branche, CL: Help your needy patients get free medication. Medical Economics [online, September 20, 1999]: *http://me.pdr.net/me/psrecord.htm*.

Darby Drug Company: *www.darbydrug.com*.

Drug Enforcement Administration: *www.DEAdiversions.usdoj.gov, www. deadiversion.usdoj.gov/drugreg/practitioners/index.html*, or 1-800-882-9539.

Fitzgerald Health Education Associates, Pharmacology Updates Seminars and Home Study Programs: 1-800-927-5380.

Florida Infusion, prescription medication sales: *www.floridainfusion.com* or 727-942-1829.

Kraft Pharmaceuticals, prescription medication sales: 1-800-887-5155.

Lowes, R: (2000, June 5). Are online pharmacies good for your patients—and for you? Medical Economics [online, June 5, 2000]: *http://www.pdr.net/ memag/public.htm?path=docs/060500/article5html*.

Marshall, A: Prescription fraud scam thwarted by officials. Clinician News (January)46:11, 2001.

Narcessian, EJ: Opioid therapy documentation kit. Purdue Pharma, Norwalk, CT, 1999.

Pearson, L: Annual update of how each state stands on legislative issues affecting advanced nursing practice. The Nurse Practitioner (January)25:16–68, 2000.

Pearson, L: Nurse Practitioner's Drug Handbook. Springhouse, Philadelphia, 2000.

Pharmaceutical Research and Manufacturers of America: *www.phrma.org/patients*.

Physicians Total Care, automated medication dispensing system: *www.physianstotalcare.com*.

Poole Arcangelo, V: Pharmacotherapeutics for Advanced Practice. Lippincott, New York, 2001.

Pyxis, automated medication dispensing system: *www.pyxis.com*.

Rxassist, *www.rxassist.org*.

Triple I Prescription Pads: P.O. Box 7431, West Trenton, NJ, 08628, or 1-800-969-7237.

Wynne, A, et al: Pharmacotherapeutics for Nurse Practitioner Prescribers. FA Davis, Philadelphia, 2001.

References

1. Chesanow, N: Your ticket to fast, flawless prescribing. Medical Economics [online, October 23, 2000]: *http://me.pdr.net/me/psrecord.htm*.

N O T E S

Chapter 10

Medical Records: How Do I Set Up My Charts?

" Good order is the foundation of all good things "

Edmund Burke

MEDICAL RECORDS

The *medical record* or *patient record* is a critical medium of communication, in both patient care and defending malpractice claims. Proper organization and handling of the medical record is imperative in providing optimal health care. The quality of the medical record is a critical factor in efforts to prevent malpractice losses. Deficiencies in documentation can have incredible consequences in leading to patient injuries, filing of claims, and defense of claims.

Basics that must be included in the documentation for every patient visit include the following:

- Patient's name, date of visit, and nurse practitioner's name
- Chief complaint
- Exam findings
- Test results
- Assessment
- Prescriptions written and injections given
- Plan
- Advice and instructions
- Time of return visit
- Signature of nurse practitioner

All entries should be written in ink, dated, and signed. All entries should be done as soon as possible. If an error is made while creating the documentation, then a single line should be drawn through the error and initialed and the correct information should be inserted. Missed or cancelled appointments should be documented in the patient's chart. All conversations must be documented. If you are serving as a preceptor for a nurse practitioner student, do not allow the student to write in the patient's chart. Documentation by a student—even if you sign it—is not acceptable documentation for Medicare. Therefore, the other insurers probably find it unacceptable too.

The importance of good record keeping cannot be overemphasized. Now is the time to fine-tune your documentation practices and make them the best possible. What are good records? Good records are accurate, comprehensive, legible, objective, timely, and unaltered.

DESIGNING PATIENT RECORDS

Well-designed forms can simplify thorough documentation of a complete history and physical examination. Designing your patient chart can be a lot of fun. You now have the chance to design the chart components the way you want them to be. With your past experience, you know what is important for you to document in your exams. The chart should hold a chronological record of the patient's encounters with the providers of the office. Design your forms so you can use them quickly while still documenting clearly and completely. Another provider should be able to pick up a chart and truly understand what is going on with that patient without having to ask a lot of questions. Preprinted patient record sheets are available from some specialty organizations as well as from health-care printing and supply companies (SYCOM 1-800-356-8141).

If you would like to create your own patient record sheets, it is easily done with a little research and good computer skills. Some of the benefits of creating your own forms are that you can modify them easily in the future, they are specific for your practice, and it may be more cost-effective to create them and have them copied as you need them. Remember, every sheet of paper in the patient's chart should include the patient's name and be fastened into the chart folder.

Another option is to purchase the *Medical Practice Forms Book & CD-ROM* (1-800-MEDSHOP), which can be customized for your practice. This book contains 130 camera-ready, tear-out forms on both paper and CD-ROM. It has chapters on business, insurance, managed care, clinical, personnel, marketing, management, data tracking, capitation, contract review, medical records, administration, and compensation.

FAMILY AND PERSONAL HISTORY

You can start by designing the patient's past medical, family, and social history sheet. This is usually completed by the patient and then reviewed with the patient by the health-care provider. Figure 10-1 outlines the basics; you may want to make modifications. On the flip side of the Family and Personal Health History form, you may want to add more questions related to your specific type of practice (e.g., menstrual, pregnancy, sexual history).

PATIENT DATA SHEET

Next, design the Patient Data Sheet, sometimes called the "welcome form." This is the form that the patient completes on his or her first visit that contains the patient's contact and insurance information (Fig. 10-2). You may want to include questions that will give you insight to the growth of your practice, such as "Where did you first learn about our practice?" Think about statistics you may want to gather about your patient base.

The patient should update the Family and Personal Health History and the Patient Data Sheet regularly. You need to have the most current information about the patient on hand. You may want to include a place for the patient to write in an e-mail address for future correspondence and marketing efforts.

PHYSICAL EXAM RECORD

The Physical Exam Record should include a place to document everything you do during your exams (Fig. 10-3). There should be space to write in any additional notes. When creating this form, remember the saying "If it isn't documented, it wasn't done." Include every aspect of the exam. Using the traditional SOAP (suggestive, objective, assessment, and plan) format may help you with organization. Include any referrals made and the time when the patient should return to your office. The signature of the nurse practitioner is required as well.

CONSENT FOR EXAMINATION

Some practices require the patient to sign a Consent for Examination (Fig. 10-4). It is not a bad idea for a nurse practitioner in independent practice to implement this form. This takes away the opportunity for a claim that you misrepresented yourself as a doctor. Take some time and think about what is important for you and your practice to know and document. Other consent forms can easily be created, but be very careful to include the required information.

PRESCRIPTION RECORD

It is good practice to keep a prescription record in the back of the chart (Fig. 10-5). It is very helpful to be able to flip to one page in the chart for reference of which prescriptions you have written for that patient. This comes in handy when the pharmacy or other providers call. Instead of having to dig through pages of notes to figure out what was written, you can keep a running log. You may want to have this printed on a color of paper specific for this form so you can locate it quickly.

PROGRESS NOTES

Progress Notes are easily created (Fig. 10-6). Use the Progress Notes to document every telephone call to and from the patient. You should also document whether the patient misses or cancels an appointment. Procedures and patient visits can be documented on this form as well.

PATIENT INTERVIEW SHEET

The Patient Interview Sheet works well if you have a medical office assistant or nurse working with you (Fig. 10-7). They can complete the initial interview with the patient and document it on the top half of the form. The bottom half is completed by the nurse practitioner. This is used for documenting patient communication and education.

RECORDS RELEASE FORM

Records Release Forms (Fig. 10-8) can be used for obtaining medical records from other providers or for forwarding records to another provider. You must have the patient's signature for the release of records.

SPECIAL PROCEDURES

If you perform office procedures, you can create specific documentation forms for those procedures (e.g., colposcopy, Norplant insertion (Fig. 10-9), intrauterine device insertion). You want to make the form easy for you to document quickly and completely.

CONSENT FORM

Before the performance of any procedure the patient and the health care provider must discuss the reason for the procedure, treatment options, and possible complications for having and for not having the procedure done. You can create your own consent forms specifically for the procedures you perform. If you are prescribing a medication that could have significant side effects, you may want to consider designing a consent form specifically for that medication protocol (see Figure 10–10). Consent forms should not be taken lightly; research what is required in the state law regarding "Informed Consent" and use it while creating your own forms.

FOLLOW-UP SYSTEMS

Plan how you would like your staff to handle test results. It is the nurse practitioner's responsibility to ensure that the patient receives and understands his or her test results. Devise a "tickler" system or log for tests ordered, consultations, and referrals. You want to make sure that what you want to get done is done in a timely fashion. Patients should be notified by the nurse practitioner—not the office staff—of any positive results. Be sure to document the conversation with the date, time, recommendations, and your signature.

Keep a running file of patients whom you are concerned about and call them back in a day or two to check on their progress or to share test results. The telephone call reinforces to the patient that you care and that you are working toward their best health.

MISSING CHARTS

Losing a chart can be a nightmare! Plan ahead and make office policy to reduce the chances of losing charts. Never let the original chart be removed from the office building. It may be tempting to carry home charts if you are behind in documenting, but don't do it. If you have this strict policy, you should never truly lose a chart. Charts should be pulled the day before the scheduled appointment and put in order at the front desk for when the patients check in the next day.

Commit yourself to completing all documentation and telephone calls before you leave for the day. If you must leave charts on your desk, have a specific area for charts only. Don't let them get mixed up with your mail and journals.

RELEASE OF RECORDS AND INFORMATION

You must establish firm rules for your staff regarding the release of medical records and information. The systems you develop should protect you and your practice against charges of breach of confidentiality and to guarantee that the records are available at any time. Before releasing any records or information, you must have a Records Release Form signed by the patient or his or her designee within the past 6 months. Be sure to release only that information that is authorized by the patient. Patients may want only certain parts of their record released. Never release the original record—release copies only. The same goes for x-ray films and findings—release only copies, never send the originals. Many states allow health-care providers to charge for copies of records that are requested from an insurance company or attorney's office ($2–$3 per page is common).

FAXING MEDICAL RECORDS

Patient confidentiality must be considered when designing your office policy on faxing patient records. You should have your fax cover sheet reviewed by your attorney to ensure proper confidentiality wording. You should make contact with the receiving office before and after faxing the record. Be sure to document the name of whom you spoke with at the receiving provider's office in the patient's chart. If your fax machine can print a confirmation of the fax sent, then keep the confirmation in the patient's chart.

STORAGE OF MEDICAL RECORDS

Think about where you will store your patient records. They should be close to the front desk for easy access when making appointments and telephone calls. Mark the charts with a sticker indicating what year the patient was last seen and update the stickers accordingly. That makes purging old charts easier. When you start having space problems for chart storage, you may want to remove charts of patients who haven't been seen in the past 5 years. You still need access to the charts, but they don't have to be in the front office. Whether you devise an alphabetical or numerical filing system, colored stickers with letters or numbers helps with filing and retrieval of charts.

There are specific state laws regarding the ownership and control of patient records. The statutes outline the laws for releasing and disposition of records in the event of the practitioner's death, termination of practice, or relocation.

ELECTRONIC MEDICAL RECORDS SYSTEMS

There are definitely some benefits to electronic medical records (EMR) systems. The reduction in errors is number one. Can you imagine no missing charts? No illegible handwriting? Many practices are implementing EMR systems. An ideal system gives the provider the choice between typing, pointing and clicking with a mouse, and voice recognition. Some programs include scheduling and billing capabilities. Some generate prescriptions and alert the provider of possible drug interactions. Some track patient's health maintenance services and give reminders of when the patient is due to be seen next. To implement an EMR system into your practice is an expensive project that may best be delayed until after you have been in practice for several years.

SUGGESTIONS AND TIPS FROM WOMEN'S HEALTH WATCH, INC.

- Different colored paper was used for the different forms at Women's Health Watch, making the forms easy to find. You may want to have your forms copied onto colored paper for quick reference.

- A computer programmer can design a template for your computer if you want to have your exam forms in your computer. This may speed up your documentation significantly.

PERSONAL ANECDOTE

I keep a 5- by 7-inch journal on my desk. I record every patient whom I am concerned about who will need follow-up. If the patient has an abnormal Pap smear, I keep her name in the journal until the case is resolved. If the patient needs an appointment in 3 months or a procedure done, I keep her name in the log. I believe that ultimately I—not my office staff—am responsible for the patient's care.

Resources

Borglum, K, and Cate, D: Medical Practice Forms Book. McGraw Hill, Santa Rosa, CA, 2001.

Carter, JH: Electronic medical records: A guide for clinicians and administrators. American College of Physicians, Philadelphia, 2001.

Lippman, H: Re-engineering your practice: Never lose a chart again. Medical Economics Magazine [online, July 24, 2000]: *http://www.pdr.net/memag/ public.htm?path=docs/article3.html.*

Lowes, R: Switching from paper to computerized charts. Medical Economics Magazine [online, May 24, 1999]: *http://www.pdr.net/memag/ static.htm?path=docs/052499/article2.html.*

Powers, J, et al: Forms facilitating primary care documentation. The Nurse Practitioner (November) 25, 40–49, 2000.

Starr, DS: When a lawyer calls for information. The Clinical Advisor (March) 12:111, 2000.

SYCOM Healthcare: 1-800-356-8141.

Figure 10–1   Family and Personal History

Name _____ Age _____ Birth Date _____ Today's Date _____

Occupation _____ Last Physical Exam Date _____ Telephone _____

Family History:	Yes	No
Alcoholism	☐	☐
Alllergies	☐	☐
Asthma	☐	☐
Arthritis	☐	☐
Anemia	☐	☐
Birth Defects	☐	☐
Bleeding Tendencies	☐	☐
Cancer, tumor	☐	☐
Colitis	☐	☐
Congenital Heart	☐	☐
Diabetes	☐	☐
Emphysema	☐	☐
Epilepsy	☐	☐
Glaucoma	☐	☐
Goiter	☐	☐
Hay Fever	☐	☐
Heart Attack	☐	☐
Heart Disease	☐	☐
High Blood Pressure	☐	☐
Kidney Disease	☐	☐
Leukemia	☐	☐
Liver Disease	☐	☐
Mental Illness	☐	☐
Migraine	☐	☐
Nervous Breakdown	☐	☐
Obesity	☐	☐
Rheumatism	☐	☐
Rheumatic Fever	☐	☐
Sickle Cell Anemia	☐	☐
Stomach Ulcer	☐	☐
Stroke	☐	☐
Suicide	☐	☐
Tuberculosis	☐	☐

Family Members:	Living	Deceased
Father	☐	☐
Mother	☐	☐
Brother(s)	☐	☐
Sister(s)	☐	☐

Your History	Yes	No
Operations:	☐	☐
Tonsils	☐	☐
Gallbladder	☐	☐
Stomach	☐	☐
Kidney	☐	☐
Colon	☐	☐
Thyroid	☐	☐
Hernia	☐	☐
Breast	☐	☐
Uterus	☐	☐
Ovaries	☐	☐
Prostate	☐	☐
Heart	☐	☐
Other _____		

Do You:	Yes	No	Amount per day
Smoke	☐	☐	_____
Drink Coffee/Tea/Colas	☐	☐	_____
Alcohol	☐	☐	_____
Drug use	☐	☐	_____

Immunizations:	Yes	No	Don't know
Pneumonia vaccine	☐	☐	☐
Tetanus	☐	☐	☐
Booster	☐	☐	☐
Measles	☐	☐	☐
Influenza	☐	☐	☐
German Measles/Mumps	☐	☐	☐
Hepatitis A	☐	☐	☐
Hepatitis B	☐	☐	☐
Other	☐	☐	☐

When was your last:

Mammogram? _____

Pap Smear? _____

Chest X-ray? _____

Other X-ray or test? _____

Figure 10-2 Patient Data Sheet

WELCOME TO
WOMEN'S HEALTH WATCH, INC.

Name: _____ Birth date: _____ Age: _____ Marital Status: _____

Address: _____ City: _____ State: _____ Zip: _____

Home Phone #: _____ Work Phone #: _____ Other: _____

Social Security Number: _____ Driver's License #: _____ Occupation: _____

E-mail Address: _____

Name of Employer: _____ Address: _____ Phone #: _____

Name of Spouse: _____ Spouse's Employer: _____

Emergency Contact Name: _____ Relationship: _____

Do you have health insurance? ☐ yes ☐ no Insurance Company: _____

Subscriber name _____ Policy Number _____

If no, how do you intend to pay? ☐ Cash ☐ Check ☐ Credit Card ☐ Medicaid ☐ Medicare

Medicaid or Medicare number: _____

How did you learn about Women's Health Watch? _____

I authorize this office to release any information necessary to expedite insurance claims. I understand that I am responsible for all charges, regardless of insurance coverage.

Patient Signature _____ Date: _____

Pharmacy Name: _____ Phone #: _____

_____

_____

_____

_____

| **Figure 10–3** | **Physical Exam Record** |

WOMEN'S HEALTH WATCH, INC.

Patient's Name _____ Exam Date _____

Age ____ LMP _____ Height _____ Weight _____ BP _____ Hgb _____ Urine PT _____

Urine: Glucose _____ Blood _____ Protein _____ Leukocytes _____

Pregnancy History: G _____ P _____ Ab _____ Misc. _____

Current Contraception/Medication: _____

Allergies: _____

Current Complaint: _____

Physical Exam

Normal   Abnormal

☐ Thyroid _____
☐ Heart _____
☐ Lungs _____
☐ Breasts _____
☐ Abdomen _____
☐ Liver _____
☐ Extremities _____

Assessment: _____

Plan: _____

_____

_____

Pelvic Exam

Normal   Abnormal

☐ Vulva _____
☐ Perineum _____
☐ Vagina _____
☐ Cervix _____
☐ Uterus _____
☐ Rectum _____
☐ Adenexa _____

Labs Done

☐ Pap Smear   ☐ Urine C&S
☐ GC   ☐ Coronary Risk
☐ Chlamydia   ☐ RPR
☐ Thyroid Profile ☐ HIV
☐ Urine PT   ☐ Serum PT
☐ Other Labs:

Educational Literature

☐ OC's   ☐ HIV/STD
☐ SBE   ☐ Meds
☐ Other _____

Post Exam Instructions:

☐ Referral
☐ Counseling/Supply visit PRN
☐ Patient voices understanding of plan
☐ Patient understands that the responsibility of follow-up is her own.

Return to Office: _____ Signature _____ ARNP

Figure 10-4   **Consent for Examination Form**

WOMEN'S HEALTH WATCH, INC.
4540 N. FEDERAL HIGHWAY
FT. LAUDERDALE, FL 33308
954/776-1500

CONSENT FOR EXAMINATION

I will be seen by a nurse practitioner who has acquired advanced education, special knowledge, and skills in the evaluation, diagnosis, treatment, education, risk assessment, health promotion, case management, coordination of care, and counseling in the primary care of adults.

I, _____, hereby request that the Nurse Practitioner examine and treat me. If appropriate, suitable contraceptive drug(s), device(s), or method(s) will be supplied, fitted or inserted, re-evaluated and changed as recommended.

I realize that if tests are taken for sexually transmitted diseases that positive results of some tests must be reported to public health agencies as required by law.

Signature _____

Date _____

Witness _____

Date _____

| Figure 10–5 | Prescription Record |

WOMEN'S HEALTH WATCH, INC.						
Date	Medication	# Dispensed	Wt.	BP	Problem/Visit	Initials

Figure 10-6 Progress Note

WOMEN'S HEALTH WATCH, INC.

Progress Note

Patient's Name: _____

Date	Progress Notes

| **Figure 10-7** | **Patient Interview Sheet** |

INITIAL INTERVIEW:

Patient here today for:

Specific complaints:

Comments:

☐ Desired form of Birth Control:_____ All C.A.R.s discussed.

☐ Condoms & HIV screening discussed – Requests screening ☐ yes ☐ no.

☐ Benefits of family planning discussed.

☐ Elementary anatomy and physiology reviewed.

☐ Overview of all contraceptive options reviewed.

☐ Information on STD screening and treatments discussed.

☐ Information on what to expect during the examination discussed.

☐ Breast self-examination techniques reviewed.

☐ Pre-conceptual counseling completed.

Interviewer's Signature _____ Date _____

EXIT INTERVIEW

☐ Individual counseling completed; all questions addressed.

☐ Patient's desired method of contraception: ☐ Approved ☐ Denied

☐ Use of contraceptive method information given: ☐ Written ☐ Verbal.

☐ Medication information sheet given.

☐ C.A.R,'s and A.C.H.E.S. discussed.

☐ Nutritional counseling completed.

☐ Hygiene discussed.

☐ Smoking cessation encouraged.

☐ Informed consents given, explained and signed.

☐ Patient given telephone number for emergency use and problems.

☐ Patient instructed to call office for laboratory results.

☐ Patient instructed to return to office for specific lab testing or results.

☐ Records Release Form signed for records to be obtained from: _____

☐ _____

☐ _____

Next appointment:

☐ Annual ☐ 6 months ☐ 3 months ☐ 1 month ☐ 2 weeks ☐ 1 week ☐ At next menses

☐ Other

Examiner's Signature _____ ARNP Date _____

| Figure 10-8 | Records Release Form |

WOMEN'S HEALTH WATCH, INC.
AUTHORIZATION FOR RELEASE OF CONFIDENTIAL MEDICAL RECORDS

Patient Name _____ D.O.B. _____

I hereby authorize: _____

_____

_____

_____

to release a summary or photocopy of my medical records to:

_____

_____

_____

Patient Signature: _____ Date _____

Witness Signature: _____ Date _____

Note: This authorization is not valid after six months from date signed.

WOMEN'S HEALTH WATCH, INC.
4540 N. FEDERAL HIGHWAY
FT. LAUDERDALE, FL 33308
954/776-1500

Figure 10-9	Special Procedures

WOMEN'S HEALTH WATCH, INC.
NORPLANT INSERTION

Name _____ Date _____ L.M.P. _____

Consent signed ☐ Yes ☐ No   Pregnancy Test ☐ Positive ☐ Negative

Lot # _____

Procedure:

    ☐ Right Arm   ☐ Left Arm

The patient was positioned supine with her arm above her head with elbow flexed. Using the NORPLANT template the arm was marked with a skin marker. The area of insertion—8–10 cm above the elbow crease in the inside of the upper arm—was prepped and draped with sterile drapes. 5cc of 1% Lidocaine plain was injected just beneath the skin in fan-like channels 15 degrees apart. A small incision was made with a #11 blade. The trocar was inserted with the bevel up. Following the NORPLANT template markings 6 NORPLANT capsules were inserted in the same plane in the fan shape using the obturator. Pressure was applied to the incision site. No excessive bleeding or hematomas noted. The edges of the incision were approximated and two Steri-strips were applied for closure. Pressure dressing applied.

Reviewed the following patient instructions and the patient verbalized an understanding of post-op care.

Patient Instructions:

- Keep pressure dressing on for 24 hours
- Keep area clean and dry for the next 3 days
- Remove Steri-strips toward the center in 3 days
- Apply ice as needed for swelling and bleeding
- Over the counter antiinflamatory as needed for pain
- Return to office in 2 weeks for arm check
- Return to the office in 3 months for menstrual check
- Call the office with any questions or concerns
- RTO by 5 year insertion anniversary for removal

Patient tolerated _____

Postoperative care sheet _____

Comments: _____

_____
Signature

Figure 10–10   **Consent Form**

EMERGENCY CONTRACEPTIVE PILLS

I have read and understand the material given to me about Emergency Contraceptive Pills. I understand that Emergency Contraceptive Pills are **definitely not** 100% effective. In spite of this, I wish to try to prevent pregnancy at this time by using Emergency Contraceptive Pills. I understand that the risk of development of birth defects in the fetus is unknown and that if this treatment fails I must accept this risk should I decide to continue with the pregnancy. I understand that I cannot take Emergency Contraceptive Pills if I have had or currently have:

- Blood clots in the veins

- Serious liver disease

- Inflammation of the veins

- Unexplained vaginal bleeding

- Any suspicions of cancer of the breast or reproductive organs

- An already established pregnancy

I understand that if I see a clinician for any reason before my next period, I should tell him/her that I have taken Emergency Contraceptive Pills. I understand that I should expect my period within 2–3 weeks and I agree to have a pregnancy test if it has not occurred within that time. I have given an accurate and complete history. No guarantee or assurance has been made to me as to the results of this treatment.

Signature of patient: _____

Date: _____

Signature of witness: _____

Date: _____

N O T E S

Chapter 11

Marketing Yourself and Your Practice: How Do I Get the Word Out?

" Nothing happens by itself...it all will come your way, once you understand that you have to make it come your way by your own exertions "

Ben Stein

There is an old saying "If you don't toot your own horn—who will?" Learning to successfully market yourself and your practice can enhance not only your career but also your self-esteem. What is marketing? Marketing encompasses everything that you and your staff do to promote your practice. Marketing begins the moment that you start thinking about opening an independent practice and continues until you discontinue practicing within that practice. Marketing includes many aspects of your business such as:

- The name, logo, and mission of your practice
- The determination of your services and products you will provide
- The way you plan to deliver those services and products
- The location of your business
- The advertising and public relations for your practice
- The training of you and your staff
- Planning the growth of your practice
- Determining how you will solve problems
- Planning how you will be following up with your current and potential patients and much, much more.

Marketing can be a complex process; however, you can keep it simple, fun, and inexpensive, and still be successful. Promoting your business requires all of the means and methods at your disposal in persuading potential patients to call your office. This can be realized through networking, advertising, publicity, public relations, special promotions, marketing materials, and client services and support.

The basic goals of your promotions should be to:

■ Let potential clients know who you are and what you are offering.

■ Let them know why they may need or want your services and products.

■ Let them know why they should come to you rather than someone else offering similar services and products.

To market your practice effectively, you must know who your potential patients are, where your potential patients are, and what is the best way to advertise to them. This planning is an ongoing process that should be evaluated and revised on a regular basis. To make your practice successful, you must always be thinking about future marketing strategies. Pay attention to what works—in other words, what efforts are bringing patients in your door.

Since marketing is an ongoing activity, never let a day pass without working on your marketing. Some business people actually schedule a certain amount of time in their daily schedule to work on promoting their businesses. Not a bad idea.

CREATING A MARKETING PLAN

Research and planning are fundamental in creating a strong business. Designing a strong marketing plan helps you organize a clear roadmap for your marketing efforts. If done properly, you will know exactly where and when to spend your advertising money and efforts. You will be creating a "care plan" to follow to help you identify and realize your goals. Marketing is an essential part of your business operations. Your marketing efforts may determine the success of your practice.

Your marketing plan will contain valuable information about your practice's services, products, marketing objectives, and strategies, as well as how you will measure your marketing successes. The marketing plan is also a section of your business plan. If you are attempting to attain financing for your practice, this marketing plan will be closely scrutinized. Ideally, the marketing plan is created before launching a business. However, if you have already launched your practice, it is not too late to develop a good marketing plan.

Marketing encompasses all of your activities from your initial research to the final delivery of service to your patients. Marketing basically looks at your products and services, price (or charges), promotion (how you let future patients know your services are available), and placement factors (where your advertising is focused). These are considered the "4 P's of marketing." Advertising is just one component of marketing—marketing is the overall strategy to promote your practice.

The objective of all new businesses should be to provide clients with services or products that they want or need. The main goal of your marketing plan is to present your services and products in such a way that your prospective clients will be encouraged to call your office and schedule an appointment to utilize those services and products.

Marketing plans usually cover marketing activities during a predetermined time span, usually 6 or 12 months. With this plan, you can estimate the costs, plan your activities, and document your successes. This plan should be updated on a regular basis; a quarterly review is recommended to keep up with changes in your practice and the market. If you have started a business plan, the first activities will be easier for you.

Before you start writing your marketing plan, you must have identified your services and products along with their features and benefits. You must have a clear idea as to who you anticipate your patients will be (this is your "target market"). You must have an idea how much you will be charging for your services and products. You must have decided on what types of credit policies you will have. You must assess your competition, their services, and their charges. You need to identify how your services are different and needed in the community. And lastly, how do you intend to attract new patients to your new practice?

Listing your services and products can help you decide what should be included in your advertising. Determining your target market will help in identifying what media sources will reach your target best. If possible, you should identify your target market by age, gender, profession, income level, educational level, and residence. This may change over the years.

Creating a "marketing calendar" can give you a quick-view reference for your past and future marketing efforts (Fig. 11–1). You will want to see as many marketing vehicles represented on your calendar as possible. The calendar helps you schedule your yearly marketing efforts and expenses. Most marketing calendars are designed using 52 weeks so you can have a good overview. Things to be included on this calendar are not only print and radio advertisements, but also your networking, public relations, and any other promotional venue. Include the time the advertisement is run, the copy deadline, and the costs (both estimated and actual).

If you can compare your charges against the competition's, you may be able to identify a specific area of your practice to promote. Brainstorming with friends, family, employees, and colleagues may lead to advertising venues you have not previously considered. Take notes when discussing advertising options with others. If the same new idea comes from more than one source, do yourself and your practice a favor and check it out. There are several potential formats for your marketing plan. You can even design your own. As long as you plan, implement your plan, and then evaluate your efforts, you are on the right track. Sample formats are provided in Boxes 11–1 and 11–2.

Your marketing plan should be designed to reach existing patients, potential new patients, hospitals, payers, referring physicians, and the community at

| Figure 11-1 | Marketing Calendar Worksheet |

Weeks of	Marketing Focus	Length	Copy Deadline	Media	Estimated Costs	Actual Costs
Eg: 9/20-10/4	New service (Sclerotherapy)	3 weeks	9/5	Chronicle (Newspaper)	$1750	$1925

Box 11–1
Formal Marketing Plan Outline

I. Executive Summary
  A. Description of your practice (services and products).
  B. Mission statement.
  C. Management team.
  D. Marketing goals and objectives.
II. Current Situation
  A. Describe current or planned location.
  B. Describe your target market.
  C. Brief competitor and issues analysis.
III. Competitor and Issues Analysis
  A. Detailed information about competitors.
  B. List key business issues and challenges.
IV. Marketing Objectives: List marketing objectives with timeframes.
V. Marketing Strategy
  A. Describe your services and products in detail.
  B. List your prices and payment policies.
  C. Describe your promotional tools.
VI. Action Programs: List your marketing "to do" list (what and when).
VII. Budget: List the costs of each of the marketing activities planned.
VIII. Measurements: List how you will measure meeting your goals.
IX. Supporting Documents: Include resumes, collateral materials, market research, spreadsheets.

Adapted from Marketing Plan Components; A Quick Review: *www.sba.gov.*

large. Your marketing strategy includes the promotion plan, which outlines the tools or tactics you will be using to attain your marketing goals. The basic components of the promotion plan include:

- Description or listing of promotional tactics
- Estimated costs for the promotional efforts
- Description of how the promotional tactics will help you attain your marketing goals

To complete this portion of the marketing plan you must do your research. Learning more about your target market and the competition will certainly give you more good information. Take some time and really think about the most efficient (time and cost) way of getting your target market in your front door. Try to put yourself in your target market's shoes; for example, don't waste money on newspaper ads if your clientele doesn't read the newspaper.

Promotional tools to include in your plan include your:

- Marketing collateral (printed materials)
- Promotional activities (trade shows, coupons, novelties)

Box 11–2
Informal Marketing Plan Outline

Long-term goals
A.
B.
C.
Short-term goals
A.
B.
C.
Describe your target market (e.g., age, gender, payment method).

Describe your target market's needs (what you will provide them).

List your strengths, weakness, and opportunities.

List your competition's strengths, weaknesses, and opportunities.

List your competitive strategies to meet goals.

Promotional plan.

Marketing and advertising budget.

Marketing timetable.

Scheduled date for review of marketing efforts.

- Public speaking and conferences
- Publications (newsletters, journals, books)
- Media relations campaigns (how you are going to keep in touch with the media)
- Advertising (print, direct mail, television, radio)

Estimate the cost for the marketing collateral and promotional activities. This will help you set a realistic budget for marketing your new practice. Take notes throughout the year so when it comes time to update your marketing plan you have specific costs, comments, and responses regarding the different avenues.

Be sure to compare your marketing strategy against your marketing objectives. Remember, your objectives must be measurable, attainable, and support the practice's vision and mission. A marketing objective may be to distribute a finite number of your brochures during a certain amount of time (e.g., 500 brochures in 3 months) or maybe attend five networking events every month. Again, really think about your target market and how you can reach them. Maybe handing out fliers with coupons at the flea market may be more appropriate than hosting a black tie gala event!

The Action Plan is a list of the important details of how and when you are going to complete your marketing objectives. If you have included on your marketing strategy that you will network at professional organization meetings, then list the meeting dates, time, and locations on the Action Plan.

The budget for the marketing plan can be designed once you have identified where you want to advertise and the costs involved. You can divide the budget into different categories, such as: collateral materials (printed materials), networking, print advertising, events, and novelties. Marketing costs vary regionally as well as with the type of media you select. There are no basic rules for deciding how much your marketing budget should be.

Marketing requires you to not only identify your target market but also to establish a competitive, unique quality to your business. If you think you need more help with marketing, attend a marketing seminar and find marketing books that make sense to you. The Small Business Association (*www.sba.gov*) can provide a lot of help with marketing your business. You can also subscribe to marketing newsletters online (e-mail *Heidi@FriskEBusiness.com*). Learn all you can about marketing—search out seminars, courses, journals, books, e-zines, and the like. The more you learn, the more you can apply, and the results can be amazing.

DEFINING YOUR NICHE

By now you have an inkling of what makes you and your practice special. You and your practice have unique characteristics. If you need to define your niche, take some time and reflect on comments that have been made to you by your patients in the past. Why do they choose to come to you? Your uniqueness may be what drives and will continue to drive patients to your practice. Take a look at what your competition is doing—identify what you can do better. Once you have identified your niche, you can fine-tune your niche market (which may also be considered your target market).

You can now create the right message, find the best media, and deliver that message to your target market. *Branding* is a term used in marketing for creating a memorable message that tells the public who you are. A couple of successful branding examples include "You deserve a break today" (McDonalds), and "Please don't squeeze the Charmin" (Charmin toilet tissues).

What do people think of when they think of your practice? Is it something like "Quality health care at affordable prices?" Or maybe it is "Progressive health care for today's woman." Some business women at a networking meeting use their branding at the end of their self introduction every month: "Never underestimate the power of the flower" (flower shop owner) and "A business with no sign is a sign of no business" (sign shop owner). They have said these clever sayings so many times that the entire group chimes in with them saying their message!

Using this *branding* concept, your goal is to *burn* a visual identity into your potential patient's mind. Whether it is from a unique and clever logo, a printed slogan, or a distinctive saying, you want your current and future patients to think of you when they are exposed to "your brand." Taking the time to think these little things through can really be worthwhile. A few questions you may want to ask yourself include:

- Does your practice's logo and slogan have the potential to evoke the desired thoughts and feelings in your target market?
- Are your printed materials eye-catching while still reflecting a professional appearance?
- How does the inside of your office look and smell? How about the outside? Windows clean, no garbage lying around? Take a look!
- Are the office hours and location appropriate for your target market?
- Do your employees treat your patients and potential patients with respect on the telephone?
- Do your employees project a professional appearance?

These are some things that may contribute or possibly work against your professional image. Your appearance also contributes to your practice's image. Anyone can wear scrubs these days. Put on a nice professional-appearing outfit and you will feel successful. People like doing business with people who look professional. Look and live the part of a professional. Dress well; be well groomed, polite, attentive, and prepared. Even when you are "off duty" and out in the community, people will recognize you. Always look good when you leave your house. Your company image is something you can't touch or feel; however, it is very important when growing your practice.

ADVISORY BOARD

Growing your business with the knowledge and expertise of others is smart business. By creating an advisory board or a brainstorming group, you can focus on increasing your business by drawing upon others' experiences. Some business organizations assist newer business owners in partnering them with successful business owners. You can create your own advisory board by developing relationships with those you feel provide you good advice.

When you put your advisory board together, choose people who have specialized knowledge that you don't have. Make a time commitment and stick with it. You may want to gather once a month or quarterly. Plan an agenda for the meeting and follow it. It is so easy to get off track and lose valuable time. Make the meetings fun so everyone will want to come to the next one. You can use this for open exchange for those involved—maybe you have knowledge that will help them with one of their concerns. Make sure that you have a policy that whatever is discussed with the group is not repeated to outsiders. Then, you can have some really interesting and valuable conversations.

There are many benefits to establishing a marketing, public relations advisory and referral team. This team can be as large or small as you wish and include whomever you think will have creative input. This team should have people who understand your practice and are interested in helping you grow your practice. Meet with "your team" on a regular basis for their input. Maybe schedule a quarterly breakfast. Be prepared to help them with their businesses as well.

Whether you decide to form a formal advisory board, to gather a casual "ideas exchange group," or simply to use your family, employees, customers, and friends, brainstorming can be invaluable. Other people see your practice from a much different perspective and may be able to give you priceless advice and ideas. Depending on your friends and family, you may want to try throwing a question out over dinner to learn their response. If the responses are helpful, take copious notes, then act on them!

PRINT NEEDS

Marketing collateral is a term used for all the printed materials used to promote your practice. It should include business cards, brochures, fliers, fact sheets, letterhead, and any other printed materials that will help promote your practice. All of your printed materials should be of the best quality possible within your budget. Promote a professional image at all times.

There are many publishing software programs available that could be helpful if you choose to design your materials yourself. Preparing your own printed material is good; however, it must have a professional finish. You may want to consider doing the rough design and layout yourself, then having it fine-tuned and professionally printed on quality paper by a printing company. No matter who is producing the materials, be sure to have several people proofread the material carefully before printing. The image you want to promote is not one of poor grammar and misspellings. Basic rule: If the material looks like a professional printer did not produce it—don't use it.

The design and layout of your printed material is important. Is it attractive and appealing? Does it contain the message you want to convey? Does it make you want to read more? A graphic designer would be helpful with creating your materials; however, with some thought you can design good materials on your own. When designing your materials, look for balance, different font types, colors, quality of paper stock, paper size, graphics, illustrations, photos, and maps.

Business Cards—Your business card is a critical marketing tool. You should be handing them out as often as possible. But first, you must design your card. Your business cards should include:

- The practice name and logo
- Your name and professional credentials
- Office address

■ Mailing address (if different from office address)

■ Telephone and fax numbers

■ Internet contact information (Website and/or e-mail address)

The design should be clever, a little different from others. You can make it unique with the design, card stock, colors, and logo. You want people to remember meeting you. Be sure the card is readable, with big enough type, clean design, and good quality print. Turn your business card into a conversation piece. An unusual design, typeface, or color scheme will help make your cards a conversation starter and memorable. You may want to consider having a fold-over card that opens into a mini brochure with a description of your practice.

Have the cards printed on quality paper (a minimum of 80 lb). Homemade cards look homemade—don't do it. Photographs on business cards may give you the look of a realtor—not the look you should be working toward! Carry your business cards wherever you go. If you are writing something down for someone, use the back of the card. That way, the person will have your number too. Some business owners choose to have Rolodex cards printed with their business card information. Magnet business cards may also be well received. They may be a bit more expensive, but how nice is it to have your business card on the refrigerators in your target market's neighborhood? Both the Rolodex and the magnet business cards give the recipient a quick reference for your contact information.

Your business card is one of the most important marketing tools you will design. The key to getting the most out of your business cards is to keep them handy. Keep them on your desk, in the reception area, in your pocket and pocketbook, and include them in all correspondence. Keep an extra supply in the glove compartment of your car and in your briefcase. Never leave home without them! Some of your friends and family may want some cards to hand out to prospective patients they speak with. Be generous. The cards are meant to be given out. They don't do you any good sitting in the box in your desk drawer!

Business Card

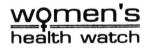

Carolyn Zaumeyer, MSN, ARNP

1735 Union Valley Road
W. Milford, NJ 07480

Phone: (954) 224-9315
(973) 728-1323
1-800-776-1519
Fax: (973) 728-9121
e-mail: whwcz@worldnet.att.net
www.independentnp.com

Figure 11-2 Appointment Card

women's
health watch
Your Next Appointment:

_____   _____
day   *date*

Time: _____
Thank You!
1234 North Weslend St. Goodtown, USA 54789

_____ (123) 456-7890 _____

Appointment cards—Your appointment cards can be printed on both sides. You could have your business card on one side, and appointment information on the other (Fig. 11–2). If you do this, it would be best to have extra business cards printed without the appointment card for networking. It could be perceived as unprofessional if you were to hand out an appointment card at a networking function. Other options for the backside of the appointment card could be a yearly calendar, your mission statement, a definition of "nurse practitioner," or health tips.

Appointment Reminder Postcards—If your practice requires the patients to return on a regular basis, the reminder postcard system could be beneficial. Design a simple postcard that you can write in the scheduled date and time of the patient's next appointment. Once the appointment is scheduled, complete the appointment information and then address the card. Write in the stamp area the ideal date to mail the card. File the card in a card file that you have set up with dividers for the 12 months. Every Monday, have your office staff mail the appropriate cards for that week. The patients appreciate this gesture as long as it isn't a confidential appointment. You may want to ask them as they are scheduling the appointment if they would like to receive a reminder postcard. If you are scheduling the appointment while the patient is there, the patient can address the card for you while you process their charges for the day.

Brochures—Before you start designing a brochure for your practice, take a few moments and think about how you will be using this collateral material. Will you be mailing it? Do you have outside locations where they can be displayed? Will you be distributing the brochures at trade shows? Does it need to fit in an envelope or in a Lucite display stand? Once you decide what the measurements of your brochure will be, you can begin sketching out the content.

The content of your brochure should clearly describe your practice. This piece should be able to sell your practice when you are not present. This should be written for the potential patient, not just to make you feel important. Information to consider including in your brochure are:

- Practice name and address
- Logo and slogan (e.g., "A Progressive Health Care Center for Today's Woman")
- Telephone and fax numbers
- Internet contact information (Website or e-mail address)
- Office hours and appointment information
- Map and/or directions to your office
- Brief biography of yourself
- Your professional photo
- Listing of professional services
- Type of payments accepted
- Anything else that is unique or special about your practice
- Languages spoken (if any other than English)

Once you have sketched out your proposed brochure, have your printer or graphic designer fine-tune the piece so it looks professional. Be sure to proofread the copy *before* it goes to print.

Once you have put the time and effort into creating your brochure—get them out! They will not benefit your practice if they stay in the box from the printer! Keep a bundle of them in your briefcase and glove compartment in your car. When you see other brochures out at networking functions, ask if you can display yours too. Whenever you speak or are out in the community marketing your practice, keep your brochures with you to help promote your practice. You may also want to include your brochure in your correspondences.

If you are fluent in another language and you want to target the community that speaks that language, you may want to have your brochure printed in that language as well. This could be a great marketing tool if you can get them distributed in the community you are targeting. You may want to check with local clinics, stores, and libraries for potential distribution points.

Having a professional brochure describing the role of the nurse practitioner in your reception area and at promotional functions can be helpful and informative. You can produce your own or purchase them. A selection of brochures may be found at *http://www.nurse.net/resources/brochure.html* or from the American Academy of Nurse Practitioners at *www.aanp.org*.

You could use your practice brochure to hand to current patients on their way out. Ask them to pass it on to a friend or family member. The simple act of explaining that your practice's growth depends on referrals can bring in many, many patients. If you have printed any other pieces with coupons, these can be given out as well. Coupons will bring in new patients.

Flyers—Usually, flyers are printed on single sheets of paper—sometimes front and back. These are great for inexpensive distribution. Fliers are frequently used to announce business openings or promote a sale, open house, or other limited time events. The headline should draw attention. Try to incorporate graphics and pictures. You can use colored copy paper or colored ink on the flyer. Make the message clear and try to motivate potential patients to call your office to schedule an appointment.

Once you have produced a nice flyer, you must get it out in the community for it to do you any good. You must always ask permission before posting or distributing flyers. Some places you may want to approach to allow you to post your flyer include:

- Schools and universities
- Student gathering places
- Faculty lounges
- Placement offices and counseling centers
- Community library
- Laundromats
- Grocery stores
- Local markets
- Subway stations
- Senior recreational facilities
- Fraternities and sororities
- Churches
- Local community clubs and organizations
- Apartment laundry rooms
- Car washes
- Hotel and motel lobbies
- Chambers of commerce
- Roller rinks and bowling alleys
- Tourist information centers
- Highway rest stops

Again, including a coupon will not only bring in new patients but will also allow you to track the success of your flyer. Knowing how many patients your flyer has brought into your practice will help you decide whether another flyer at a later time is worth the time, money, and effort spent on producing and distributing the flyer.

Stationery—A professional-appearing letterhead gets people's attention. Think about receiving a letter on nice quality paper with a professionally printed heading, compared to receiving a letter on a plain white sheet of thin, inexpensive paper. It may seem trivial, but if you want your correspondence to receive the most attention possible, give the design and printing your attention. Matching envelopes and second page sheets are a must as well.

Your letterhead should complement your business card. Use the same type, colors, and logo for your business cards, letterhead and envelopes so they all match. Your practice image should be steady and memorable. You might want to have some inexpensive white envelopes printed with your return address for mailing bills and other miscellaneous correspondence.

Fax Cover Sheets—You can design your fax cover sheet on your computer using your practice's letterhead or on plain white paper. Besides your contact information that is included on your letterhead, you will also want to include a space to write for whom the fax is intended, their fax number, the date, number of pages sent, and a place for a note. Be sure to use a large enough type that is easy to read. It is very frustrating to read a fax in which the print is too small or blurred. Depending on your state law, you may need to include a privacy statement if you are faxing medical records.

Once you have designed a fax cover sheet that includes all of the information necessary and has a professional appearance, make a lot of copies. Keep the copies close to the fax machine so it is a quick and easy process to send a fax. Be sure to file the original (or master) aside in a safe place so you will be able to reproduce it clearly in the future. Copies of copies over time become blurry and unreadable. Be sure to design your form with a confidentiality notice (Box 11–3).

Box 11–3
Sample Confidentiality Notices

Sample 1

CONFIDENTIALITY NOTICE

The information contained in this facsimile is intended only for the use of the individual named above. This information may be privileged or confidential. If you are not the intended recipient, be aware that any disclosure, copying, distribution, or use of the contents is strictly prohibited.

If you have received this transmission in error, please call (555-555-5555) to arrange for return or destruction of the transmission at our expense.

Sample 2

The information contained in this facsimile message is legally privileged and confidential information. It is intended ONLY for the use of the addressee. If the reader of this message is not the intended recipient or a duly authorized agent who is responsible for delivering the information to the intended recipient, you are hereby notified that any dissemination, distribution or photocopying of this facsimile is strictly prohibited. If you have received this facsimile in error, please notify *Facility Name* by calling (555) 555-5555 immediately and return this document to: *Facility Name* at *Facility Address*. Return postage via the U.S. Postal Service is guaranteed. Thank you.

When preparing your collateral materials, try to be creative. Use catchy slogans and eye-catching terminology. Use a bit of color when possible. Highlight the benefits of coming to your practice. Remember, your printed material represents you and your practice when you are not present. Send the best message possible.

NETWORKING

Business comes from relationships. Whether you are thinking about possibly gaining patients from colleagues or word of mouth from current patients, business comes from relationships. To quote one of the best business trainers I know, Susan Leventhal of Susan Leventhal & Associates in Ft. Lauderdale, Florida, "People need to get to know you, to like you, and to trust you. Then, business is sure to follow!" If you join a networking group, chamber of commerce, or other business group, don't expect any business to come without letting people get to know you. See Box 11–4 for the Websites of some national business networking organizations. Marketing is a personal and long-term relationship building process.

Do you classify yourself as "shy?" Now is the time to get over it. Most successful people have learned to overcome their shyness. You must not wait for

---

Box 11–4

Business Networking Organizations' National Offices

American Business Women's Association	*www.abwahq.org*
Business Women's Network	*www.bwni.com*
Business and Professional Women, USA	*www.bpwusa.org*
Chamber of Commerce	*www.chamber-of-commerce.com/search.htm*
Forum for Women Entrepreneurs	*www.fwe.org*
Latin Business Association	*www.lbausa.com*
Lions Club	*www.lionsclub.org*
National Association of Women Business Owners	*www.nawbo.org*
National Foundation for Women Business Owners	*www.nfwbo.org*
Rotary International	*www.rotary.org*
The Women's Chamber of Commerce	*www.thewomenschamber.com*
Toastmasters International	*www.toastmasters.org*
United States Hispanic Chamber of Commerce	*www.ushcc.com*
United States Small Business Administration	*www.sba.gov*
Women Incorporated	*www.womeninc.com*

people to approach you, you must train yourself to reach out and extend yourself to people. A good handshake and eye contact with a smile goes a long way in promoting yourself and your practice.

There is an art and science to mastering networking skills. You and your employees should hone networking skills. Include your employees in networking training. Encourage them to help you market your practice wherever they go. Networking develops a relationship that fosters a sense of caring and responsibility. Networking creates the opportunity for you to help one another advance your businesses. The key to successful networking is listening and learning. If you can help them, chances are that they will want to help you.

Think about how you present yourself to your patients and the community. This is critical because you *are* the business. You must exude confidence, knowledge, kindness, trust, compassion, and credibility. You need to demonstrate your expertise, trustworthiness, and concern for your patients' (or potential patients') welfare. What image would you like to see when you first meet or visit your health-care provider? Patients have many choices of whom they may entrust with their health care.

In service businesses, customers leave the business for a variety of reasons, but most of those who leave will leave because of a poor attitude by you or your employees. Try to reduce unnecessary attrition of your patient base with a "zero tolerance" policy for rudeness by your employees. Encourage and reward kindness extended by your employees. And, of course, be an excellent example. Many times, employees will mirror the attitudes of their employers.

Before setting out to "network," you should set some goals. What would you like to accomplish with your networking efforts? Whom would you like to meet who will help you reach your goals? Where can you find the people who will help you realize your goals? Can you devote a set amount of time to developing relationships with these people? How much time do you think you will need to devote to networking? What type of events would be best for you to direct your networking efforts?

Every time you meet someone, you have the opportunity to turn it into a networking situation. There are many places to use your networking skills: business organization meetings, professional organization meetings, cocktail parties, political events, charity events, social events, and more. Check the business calendar in your local newspaper for a listing of networking functions in your area. You are not limited to planned functions for networking. You can meet people and find a common interest (and bring your practice into the conversation at some point!) anywhere. From the grocery to the gym, to wherever there are people willing to talk—you may find prospective patients.

Networking success not only involves being prepared to promote your business, but also being able to listen and "connect" with others. Really listen, ask questions, and demonstrate sincere interest in others. Let them get to know you, get to like you, and get to trust you. When you meet someone new at a networking function, be sure to ask him or her for a business card. You may later think of a way this person could help you and your practice. You may call upon their expertise or even team with them in a promotional program. If you don't get the business card, it may be difficult to locate that person later. By asking for another person's card, chances are that person will also ask for yours. When passing on your card, you may be opening yourself up for great new opportunities (and possibly new patients too!).

Design a clever name tag with both your practice's name and your name and wear it to networking functions. If you have a logo, include the logo on your name tag. Be sure that the name tag is made of good quality and is durable. You and your employees should all wear name tags in the office. Include the employee name and title on the name tag. Your patients will like knowing with whom they are speaking. As a rule, when networking, you should wear your name tag on your right lapel. That way, when you lean in to shake someone's hand, it brings your name tag closer to the person's eye. The goal is to have the person read your tag, repeat your name, and remember your name.

You may consider purchasing professional lab coats and having your name and title embroidered on the left upper chest section above the pocket. The lab coat should be worn only in your office or in the hospital. People like to know the names and titles of people they are dealing with. Patients deserve to know the name and level of education of the people caring for them.

To spread the good news of your new practice, you must join professional organizations, chambers of commerce, and business networking organizations. Make the most of your efforts—arrive early, try to meet everyone in the room, and attend the social hour if there is one. Once you have other members' mailing addresses, you might want to write a letter of introduction and include your brochure, business card, and newsletter. These letters are best mailed after you have joined the organization. You don't want to appear that you are using the organization just for its mailing list.

You need to get out of your office and start introducing yourself to as many new people as possible. Identify key business and professional organizations that sound interesting to you. Go to the meetings regularly and get to know the members. You may even choose to eventually serve on a committee or even the organization's board of directors. Keep your mind on your goal to meet more and more people—not just meet them, but also impress them so that they will want to get to know you, trust you, and work with you. By getting involved, you give yourself the opportunity to be more visible—which is free advertising!

Networking can be done everywhere you go, from restaurants, to stores, to professional offices, and more. Let people know who you are, what you are, what your business is about, and how they can help you. You may be surprised at the referrals that come in once you start networking to the fullest.

Do not overlook fellow nurses and nurse practitioners as referral sources and potential patients. Be sure to let them know that their referrals are important to you. Also, find a way to support their business if possible. Even if it is a simple letter to their employer about their professional appearance and behavior, the person named in the letter will certainly appreciate it. Employers like to know that their institution is being represented well in the community.

When networking, try not to act desperate for business. Listen to others about their businesses and be ready to share positive information that will draw them to your practice. Stay focused on the conversation and bringing in business. Give the appearance of mingling—not selling. Be ready to follow up the next day with a telephone call or a note to really make your meeting memorable. Be a good conversationalist and be interesting to talk with. Part of networking is getting the other person to talk and feel comfortable. Think of some general questions to ask that will get them talking about themselves. When you meet someone, ask him or her what he or she does. Then, be prepared with a three- to four-sentence description of your work. When the other person is talking, look directly at him or her and focus on the content of the conversation.

Prepare and practice a short definition of the role of the nurse practitioner and how we differ from physicians. To help you prepare your definition, review the videotape or CD-ROM produced by the American Academy of Nurse Practitioners *www.aanp.org*. Try to keep it on a positive note; slamming physicians and their practices is sure to backfire against you and your practice. Read the local papers regularly for new marketing ideas and seminars. Keep an eye out for your competition's advertising methods.

People enjoy happy optimistic people. Optimism is one of the few common characteristics of successful entrepreneurs. Your attitude is under your control. People do not search out people who present a down or depressed look—they are drawn to smiling, happy people. Keep abreast of the local business news; you may be able to work the news into your conversations. Also, if you keep current, you may recognize some of the movers and shakers in the business community who may be able to help you grow your business. Networking can be very rewarding and a lot of fun!

Be careful not to inadvertently "turn-off" the person you are speaking with. Some basic rules include:

1. Don't ramble on and on. Be concise but not short. Don't tell them more than they want to know.

2. Be careful not to brag. Nobody likes a braggart. Watch out for the "I's" in your conversation.

3. Do not ask a professional for free advice. Ask if you can call and schedule a consultation. You have probably been a victim of this and it just isn't right.

4. Do not let your mind and eyes wander when you are being spoken to. Pay attention to your conversation.

5. Do not interrupt or finish the sentences of the person speaking to you.

6. Never use curse words or bigoted comments. Ever.

7. Do not do all of the speaking; let the other person talk, so they will feel good about the interaction.

8. Do not force your business card on anyone. If the appropriate time comes up in conversation to share your card, do so, then, reciprocate by asking for the other person's. You can learn a lot about people by looking at their business card. It also gives you more information for conversation.

9. Do not go to a networking function without freshening your breath! Mouthwash, toothpaste, breath mints, and even gum can help you get a fresh start. Of course, remove the gum from your mouth before you enter the event.

10. Do not give a weak or too strong handshake. Practice with friends or family. Be careful not to squeeze an older person's hand too hard; it may hurt. Then again, don't give the limp "dead fish" handshake either.

When you receive a business card from someone, write a note to yourself on the back of the card about the person and his or her business after you leave the function. You may want to add that person to your database for your newsletter and other mailings. Keep the cards—it may be 6 months later when you want or need to contact them and you will be able to find their contact information easily.

ADVERTISEMENTS

You cannot depend on "word of mouth" advertising only. You must get the word out that you are in practice in every way possible. The basics include the signage, telephone directories, Internet Websites, newspapers, telephone, radio, and direct mailings.

When contacting the media for advertising information, ask for a *rate sheet*. This rate sheet gives prices for the different advertising options for that media source. Don't be afraid to bargain on the prices. Many times the media can be flexible, especially for a new small business. Make an offer you can afford, and you may be pleasantly surprised. Also ask about deadlines for submission and if the media source will complete the artwork for any printing. You should lay out the basic information contained in the advertisement, and the media source will usually fine-tune the ad to give it a professional look.

If you are interested in possibly advertising in larger publications (major magazines and newspapers) that have "remnant space" (space that hasn't been sold), contact the media source or get in touch with Media Networks, Inc., at 1-800-225-3457. Media Networks is a national company that provides a free rate book for placing remnant advertisements—you may have a great opportunity waiting for you.

Put together a worksheet that will work for you when gathering the costs of your different marketing vehicles so you will be able to clearly make a plan within your marketing budget (Fig. 11–3).

Figure 11–3	Marketing Methods Cost Estimations Worksheet

Marketing Method	Quantity	Designer	Source	Estimated Cost	Time to Produce	Actual Costs
Business Cards						
Appointment Cards						
Postcards						
Brochures						
Flyers						
Stationery						
Fax Cover Sheet						
Networking						
Organization Membership Fees						
Signage						
Telephone Directories						
Internet and Website						
Newspaper						
Radio						
Television						
Direct Mail						
Other Advertising Venues						
Trade Show Exhibits						
Newsletters						
E-zines						
Grand Opening						
Comment Cards						
Novelties						
Contests						

Signage—Properly crafted, freestanding, brightly lit signs can be the best advertising method possible. Including signs on all doors can also be beneficial. Be sure the name of the practice and the telephone number is readable from the road. Before designing your signs, take a few moments and drive around the area. Assess the signs for readability. What signs jump out at you and why? Is it the size or type of lettering? Is it the colors they used? Is it the location? Keep your signs simple, clear, and classy.

Assess the parking lot entrance and exit. Do you need to have signs printed to avoid confusion? Can your new patients easily find your office suite from the parking lot or is additional signage necessary?

Telephone Directories—When starting your practice, one of the best marketing tools to consider is the telephone directory. Contact the telephone company to locate a sales representative. The representative can tell you the deadline date for advertisement placement in the next printing of the directory. The representative can also provide the different options of size and location of the advertisements. There are several companies now producing telephone directories. Be sure you are dealing with the one that will give you the most exposure.

Take a few minutes and review the directory you are considering. What categories would be appropriate for your advertisements? What is the minimum size that you think would be effective? Do you need to use color print? Be sure to review your competitor's advertisements. Consider the competition's ads when designing your own. The advertisement rates may help you with your decisions. Directory advertisement may seem costly; however, it may be a huge mistake not to advertise in the directory.

There are basically three types of advertisements in the telephone directories: Regular listings, informational listings, and display ads. The regular listings are the small text lines that most businesses have in the general listings. Informational listings are the ones in columns with boxes around them with more information and customization available. Display ads are the larger ads outside of the column. Whatever type you decide is appropriate for your practice, try to get exposure in as many categories as possible.

Many people, especially those without insurance coverage, shop for providers in the telephone directory. The patient who typically refers to the telephone directory is one who is usually new to the community or is in search of a new health-care provider. Many patients like to find specialists through the directory, rather than asking their primary care provider. Some of the directory users are looking for their existing provider's telephone number to schedule an appointment.

When people open a directory, they usually go to the section that best represents their needs. They look for the specialty, location, familiar name, or attractive image. They may even be looking for a provider of a certain gender or ethnicity. The space of the advertisement should be designed with care. You want to provide a good overview of your services, hours, insurance accepted, and languages spoken. The directory usually provides a free design service for your advertisement. Be sure to proofread the copy carefully before approving the final design. You can design the advertisement yourself and give it to the representative, but insist on seeing the ad before it goes to print. If there is an error in the copy, you may have to live with it for a year until the next directory is printed. If you are not sure of some of the details, such as your office hours, do not include them. Make sure that whatever you print in the ad will still be correct in 1 year's time. Keep a copy of the proof you have approved on file.

The nationally sanctioned heading for telephone directories is *Nurse—Practitioners*, however, you should write a letter to your local yellow page provider stating that the heading should really be *Nurse Practitioners*. An example of the letter you should send can be found at *http://www.nurse.net/media/yp.ltr.html*.

Internet—Many people are using the Internet as a directory to find a health-care provider. The Internet is a powerful marketing tool that every small business owner should consider. Designing a Website can be inexpensive and fun. If you do not want to spend your time developing the site, there are many Website developers willing to help you for a fee. Possibly a friend or family member would do it for free. A Website can be a great marketing tool. You can include a lot of material on a simple three-page Website. Your patients (and possibly future patients) may also be able to contact you by e-mail through the Website. Many people will then perceive you as being contemporary, progressive, and in touch with the public.

Try to get a catchy domain name that is easy to remember. You can search and register your domain name with many companies, for example, VeriSign at *http://www.netsol.com*. If you sell products in your office, you may want to offer the products for sale through your Website. CCnow (*www.ccnow.com*) or Paypal (*www.paypal.com*) can set up your order form and attach it to your Website. CCnow and Paypal can process your credit card orders. Once the order is placed, the service e-mails you the order and you can then process the order. It works very well and the fees are reasonable. Your Internet Website should be registered on the major search engines. This is an area that needs to be checked monthly. There are professionals who can do this for you or you can learn to monitor your presence on the Internet yourself. Be sure to include your Website address and e-mail address on all of your marketing materials.

If you or someone you know would like to design a basic Website for your practice, there are several Internet services programs that will walk you through the process and they are relatively inexpensive. Try *www.imagecafe.com*, which has excellent customer service and is very user friendly.

There are two excellent Websites that direct consumers directly to nurse practitioners in their area. To register yourself in the directory, go to *http://www.npclinics.com*. and *http://www.nurse.net*. These are the same Website addresses that consumers will use to find a nurse practitioner. Your practice can then be found by entering zip code, state, specialty, practitioner name, or practice name.

You may also find opportunities to advertise your practice on the Internet at different locations. Look for Websites that would be good for your practice to be included in their "Link" section. If you have seen an online newsletter (e-zine) produced by someone else, you may want to inquire about adding an advertisement section for your practice.

Newspapers—Print advertising can be a wonderful way to bring in new patients. When designing print advertisements, it is best to use different fonts, shapes, and colors to keep the reader's attention. Busier layouts many times get a better response than the more simple advertisements. Inserting a good quality photograph of yourself may be eye-catching as well. Keep in mind, however, that your main goal with your advertising piece is to motivate a prospective patient to go to the telephone to call and schedule an appointment! To do this, you may want to try to create a sense of urgency—if you are using a coupon, include an expiration date within the next month or two. Besides coupons, the word "Free" seems to motivate people too. Whether it is a free consultation, gift, or sample, people love "Free!" It is estimated that more than 75% of the American households use coupons at some point. You may want to mail coupons for savings to your regular patients once or twice a year.

Another approach could be to target your ad to one service for a particular segment of your target market. You could do a series of advertisements with the same basic layout but different features each week. Develop a strong headline for your print advertisement. Depending on your target market, you can focus your headline appropriately. Create something that will be eye-catching (e.g., "Be kind to your Valentine—get tested for Sexually Transmitted Diseases Today!"). Then reinforce your headline with good copy that supports the headline. End the copy by telling the reader how to respond to your advertisement: "Call 555-1234 for FREE information TODAY!" Be sure to have the telephone number printed in larger bold numbers. Keep working on new headlines and copy designed specifically for different media and audiences.

Letters to the editor are a popular section of local newspapers. They are usually limited to a specific length (usually less than 300 words) and require the letter writer's name. You should include the date and title of the article that prompted your response. Use clear and concise wording in your letter. Clearly state your point. Be sure your letter is well written without spelling and grammatical errors, otherwise it may never get published. If your letter is in response to a specific article, your letter should arrive within 1 week of the original printing of the article.

Over the past few years, "advertorials" have been used more and more for health-care providers. Advertorials are advertisements that are written to either look like an editorial column in the newspaper or sound like a patient's testimonial to your services on the radio. These advertorials can be quite successful with both the newspaper and the radio. Another format that has become popular is writing the ad to appear like a health-care question and answer column: "Dear Nurse Practitioner, I feel dizzy everyday at 10:00 a.m. What tests should I have to find out what is going on?" You can come up with clever questions that relate specifically to your practice and highlight the services you would like to promote.

Depending on your target market, you may want to investigate the different types of newspapers in your community. Whether the paper is directed to senior citizens or concert-goers, find the newspaper that will best reach your target market.

Radio and Television—It is good to investigate the costs of radio and television advertisements so you will be able to make informed choices with your advertisement budget. Most radio and television advertisement spots are expensive. You must evaluate the viewing or listening audience. You need to have the confidence that your target market will be seeing or hearing the advertisements that you are paying for. This may best be a venue to put on hold until your practice is more established and your advertising budget is higher.

Research radio talk shows for ones that have health topics. Listen to the show and call in with accurate health information that contributes to the show. Be sure to say your name and your practice's name clearly and often. When you are on the air, be sure to speak with enthusiasm and avoid speaking in a monotone. Limit your use of medical jargon and be prepared for questions. You may want to contact the radio stations to avail yourself to lead a radio talk show on health issues.

Be sure to include local radio and television stations on your media list for press releases. If you are the first nurse practitioner in independent practice in your area, you may have a good chance of being interviewed. What wonderful free press!

Direct Mail Pieces—There are several options regarding the type of direct mail you may want to use. You can use your newsletter, a postcard, letters, flyers, advertisements, brochures, and coupons. The size and shape of direct mail pieces vary but they must comply with standard mailing requirements. Direct mail pieces are usually designed and mailed out by a direct mail service company. There are many different mailing lists of addresses for you to choose from.

The effectiveness of this method of advertising for health-care providers is questionable. If you do a mailer, be sure to have a way to monitor the effectiveness of the mailing. Having a different-appearing coupon with a certain percentage or dollar amount of the patient's charges is an effective measure of the advertising program. You can target the audience of your choice by identifying your target market and describing it to the direct mail agency. You can also send different pieces to different groups. If you like the piece that has been created, ask to have extra copies printed to hand out at functions and to your patients. Keep a current list of "hot prospects" of both patients and referral sources that you would like to target with your marketing strategies.

If you are designing and mailing the direct mail piece yourself, you may want to consider or include the following:

- Design the envelope to be eye-catching and memorable. Use bright colors, graphics, photographs, and a clear message.
- Use uncomplicated language: "Save," "free," "new," "learn," "easy," and "now" all are words that make for a clear and simple message that everyone will understand.

- Sell the benefits of using your services.
- Patient testimonials may be interesting.
- Use at least two colors of ink.

If you are doing the mailing yourself, you can purchase a mailing list on disc, labels, or magnetic tapes from a list broker. Be sure to specify who is included in your target market. Make sure the list is current and has been updated within the last 3 to 6 months. The list should be guaranteed 90% to 95% deliverable. Lists may cost anywhere from $10 to more than $100 per thousand names. Before you commit to this project (or any other advertising), sketch out the proposed budget. Check with the post office for mailing rates to find the easiest and least expensive way to complete the mailing. Be sure to track this advertising method with a unique coupon so you can evaluate the success of your marketing efforts (Fig. 11–4).

Other Advertising Venues—Once your practice is up and going, you may want to consider some "nontraditional" creative marketing tactics such as:

- Advertise on bus backs and sides.
- Advertise on bus stop benches.
- Advertise on billboards.
- Write banner ads on popular Websites.
- Advertise in the classified section of newspaper.
- Use a vanity automobile license tag.
- Advertise at the movie theater.
- Advertise at the bowling alley.
- Advertise on restaurant signs and placemats.
- Create bumper stickers.
- Create calendars.
- Support or sponsor charitable events.
- Volunteer to work at charitable events.
- Sponsor an "Adopt-a-Road" area in your community to keep the roads clean. Everyone who drives by your sign will see you are doing good things for the community.
- Write educational pamphlets or a book.
- Print caps and T-shirts to give away.
- Host a public access television show.
- Write a newspaper article or column.
- Host a holiday party.
- Take an editor to lunch.
- Extend your office hours.
- Serve in a public office.

Patient's Name	Telephone Directory	Patient Referral (write name)	Provider Referral (write name)	Newspaper	Networking	Signs	Other

- Host a 5K run for a charity.
- Star in your own radio advertisement or talk show.
- Create and present an award for someone in the community.
- Locate and get published in local business directories.
- Print and distribute door hanger advertisement pieces.
- Display an exhibit at the county or state fairs.
- Get public relations training.
- Submit "health tip" articles to newspapers.
- Conduct and publish research.
- Design and promote gift certificate sales for your services.
- Develop and advertise a "help-line" for health information.
- Host an open house.
- Mentor a student.
- Host an "invitation only" event at your office.
- Add a telephone message for callers to listen to while they are on hold (*www.onhold-messages.com*).
- Cross promotions—work with other businesses that complement your practice to share advertising costs (e.g., women's health office advertising along with a beauty salon).
- Display vehicle signage.
- Hire a blimp or banner ad behind a small airplane.
- Learn from your competitors .
- Display restroom advertisements.
- Advertise on signs on airport luggage carousels.
- Advertise on roadside sandwich board signs.
- Contact your local Welcome Wagon to be included in their welcome basket.
- Display telephone booth advertisements.
- Add a 1-800 number.
- Use bulletin boards at laundromats, apartments, and grocery stores.
- Be enthusiastic.
- Market your practice to local hotels for house calls and flexible hours.
- Add your professional initials to your personal checks.
- Join or register with speaking bureaus.
- Sponsor a needy child's camp tuition.
- Sponsor a softball or baseball team.
- Request assistance from pharmaceutical and medical suppliers.

- Make up something to celebrate.
- Send birthday cards to patients (include a novelty or lotto card if possible!).
- Send thank-you cards to patients for referrals.
- Tie your advertising and promotional activities to an appropriate national health observance day, week, or month (Box 11–5).

Box 11–5

National Health Observance Calendar

Note: Contact sponsoring organization to verify dates (some change annually) and to receive free promotional materials.

January

Cervical Health Awareness Month	*www.nccc-online.org*
National Cervical Cancer Coalition	
National Glaucoma Awareness Month	*www.preventblindness.org*
Prevent Blindness America	
National Birth Defects Prevention Month	*www.modimes.org*
March of Dimes Birth Defects Foundation	
National Volunteer Blood Donor Month	*www.aabb.org*
American Association of Blood Banks	

January 20–26

Healthy Weight Week	*www.healthyweight.net*
Healthy Weight Network	

February

American Heart Month	*www.americanheart.org*
American Heart Association	
AMD/Low Vision Awareness Month	*www.preventblindness.org*
Prevent Blindness America	
National Children's Dental Health Month	*www.ada.org*
American Dental Association	
Sinus Pain Awareness Month	*www.entnet.org*
American Academy of Otolaryngology	
Wise Health Consumer Month	*www.aipm.healthy.net*
American Institute for Preventative Medicine	

February 3–9

Cardiac Rehabilitation Week	*www.aacvpr.org*
American Association of Cardiovascular and Pulmonary Rehabilitation	

February 3-9:

National Burn Awareness Week	*www.shrinershq.org*
Shriners Burn Hospital	

February 6
National Girls and Women in Sports Day
  Women's Sports Foundation

www.womenssportsfoundation
.org

February 10–16
National Child Passenger Safety
Awareness Week
  Office of Occupant Protection, National
  Highway Traffic Safety Administration

www.nhtsa.dot.gov

February 10–16
National Children of Alcoholics Week
  National Association for Children
  of Alcoholics

www.naccoa.net

February 14
National Condom Day
  American Social Health Association

www.ashastd.org

March
Mental Retardation Awareness Month
  The ARC of the United States
National Colorectal Cancer
Awareness Month
  Cancer Research Foundation of America
National Eye Donor Month
  Eye Bank Association of America
National Kidney Month
  National Kidney Foundation
National Nutrition Month
  American Dietetic Association
Workplace Eye Health and Safety Month
  Prevent Blindness America

www.thearc.org

www.preventcancer.org

www.restoresight.org

www.kidney.org

www.eatright.org/nnm/

www.preventblindness.org

March 3–9
Save Your Vision Week
  American Optometric Association

www.aoanet.org

March 4–8
National School Breakfast Week
  American School Food Service

www.asfsa.org

March 10–16
Pulmonary Rehabilitation Week
  American Association of Cardiovascular
  and Pulmonary Rehabilitation

www.aacvpr.org

March 17–23
National Poison Prevention Week
  Poison Prevention Week Council

www.cpsc.gov

March 17–23
National Inhalants and Poisons
Awareness Week   *www.inhalants.org*
 National Inhalant Prevention
 Coalition

March 24
World Tuberculosis Day   *www.aaworldhealth.org*
 American Association for World Health

March 27
American Diabetes Alert   *www.diabetes.org*
 American Diabetes Association

April
Alcohol Awareness Month   *www.ncadd.org*
 National Council on Alcoholism
 and Drug Dependence
Cancer Control Month   *www.cancer.org*
 American Cancer Society
Counseling Awareness Month   *www.counseling.org*
 American Counseling Association
Irritable Bowel Syndrome Awareness   *www.iffgd.org*
Month
 International Foundation for Functional
 Gastrointestinal Diseases
National Autism Awareness Month   *www.autism-society.org*
 Autism Society of America
National Child Abuse Prevention Month *www.calib.com/nccanch*
 National Clearinghouse on Child
 Abuse and Neglect Information
National Occupational Therapy Month *www.aota.org*
 American Occupational Therapy
 Association
National STD Awareness Month   *www.ashastd.org*
 American Social Health Association
National Youth Sports Safety Month   *www.nyssf.org*
 National Youth Sports Safety Foundation
Women's Eye Health Safety Month   *www.preventblindness.org*
 Prevent Blindness America

April 1–7
National Public Health Week   *www.apha.org*
 American Public Health Association

April 4
Kick Butts Day   *www.tobaccofreekids.org*
 National Center for Tobacco-Free Kids

April 5–7
Alcohol-Free Weekend   *www.ncadd.org*
  National Council on Alcoholism and Drug
  Dependence, Inc.

April 7
World Health Day   *www.aawhworldhealth.org*
  American Association for World Health

April 14–20
National Infants Immunization Week   *www.cdc.gov/nip*
  Centers for Disease Control
  and Prevention

April 14–20
National Minority Cancer   *www.cancernet.nci.nih.gov*
Awareness Week
  Cancer Information Service

April 21–27
National Organ and Tissue   *www.shareyourlife.org*
Donor Awareness Week
  Coalition on Donation

April 27–28
WalkAmerica   *www.modimes.org*
  March of Dimes Birth Defects Foundation

May
Asthma and Allergy Awareness Month   *www.aafa.org*
  Asthma and Allergy Foundation
  of America
Better Hearing and Speech Month   *www.asha.org*
  American Speech-Language-
  Hearing Association
Older Americans Month   *www.aoa.gov*
  Administration on Aging
Skin Cancer Awareness Month   *www.cancer.org*
  American Cancer Society
Better Sleep Month   *www.bettersleep.org*
  Better Sleep Council
Clean Air Month   *www.lungusa.org*
  American Lung Association
Correct Posture Month   *www.amerchiro.org*
  American Chiropractic Association
Hepatitis Awareness Month   *www.hepfi.org*
  Hepatitis Foundation International
Huntington's Disease   *www.hdsa.org*
Awareness Month
  Huntington's Disease Society
  of America, Inc.

Lyme Disease Awareness Month	*www.lyme.org*
Lyme Disease Foundation	
National Arthritis Month	*www.arthritis.org*
National Arthritis Foundation	
National High Blood Pressure	*www.nhlbi.nih.gov*
Education Month	
National Heart, Lung, and	
Blood Institute	
National Melanoma/Skin	*www.aad.org*
Cancer Detection	
And Prevention Month	
American Academy of Dermatology	
Mental Health Month	*www.nmha.org*
National Mental Health Association	
National Neurofibromatosis Month	*www.nf.org*
National Neurofibromatosis Foundation	
National Osteoporosis Prevention Month	*www.nof.org*
National Osteoporosis Foundation	
National Stroke Awareness Month	*www.stroke.org*
National Stroke Association	
National Teen Pregnancy	*www.advocatesforyouth.org*
Prevention Month	
Advocates for Youth	
National Trauma Awareness Month	*www.amtrauma.org*
American Trauma Society	

May 5–11

Food Allergy Awareness Week	*www.foodallergy.org*
Food Allergy and Anaphylaxis Network	

May 5–11

National SAFE KIDS Week	*www.safekids.org*
National SAFE KIDS Campaign	

May 5–11

National Suicide Awareness Week	*www.suicidology.org*
American Association of Suicidology	

May 7

Childhood Depression Awareness Day	*www.nmha.org*
National Mental Health Association	

May 8

National Anxiety Disorders Screening Day	*www.freedomfromfear.org*
National Mental Illness Screening Project	

May 12–18

National Alcohol and Other Drug Related	*www.ncadd.org*
Birth Defects Week	
National Council of Alcoholism and Drug	
Dependence	

May 12–18
National Running and Fitness Week   *www.americanrunning.org*
   American Running Association

May 13–19
National Stuttering Awareness Week   *www.stuttersfa.org*
   Stuttering Foundation of America

May 15
National Employee Health and   *www.physicalfitness.org*
Fitness Day
   National Association for Health
   and Fitness

May 19–25
National Emergency Medical   *www.acep.org*
Services Week
   American College of Emergency
   Physicians

May 25
National Missing Children's Day   *www.childfindofamerica.org*
   Child Find of America, Inc.

May 29
National Senior Health and Fitness Day   *www.fitnessday.com*
   Mature Market Resource Center

May 31
World "No Tobacco" Day   *www.aawhworldhealth.org*
   American Association for World Health

June
National Trauma Awareness Month   *www.amtrauma.org*
   American Trauma Society
National Aphasia Awareness Month   *www.aphasia.org*
   National Aphasia Association
National Scleroderma Awareness Month   *www.scleroderma.org*
   Scleroderma Foundation

June 5
National Cancer Survivors Day   *www.cancer.org*
   American Cancer Society

June 6–8
National Headache Awareness Week   *www.headaches.org*
   National Headache Foundation

June 10–16
National Men's Health Week   *www.nationalmenshealthweek*
   National Men's Foundation   *.com*

June 23–29
Helen Keller Deaf-Blind Awareness Week   *www.helenkeller.org*
   Helen Keller National Center

July
Hemochromatosis Screening   *www.hemochromatosis.org*
Awareness Month
   Hemochromatosis Foundation
Fireworks Safety Month   *www.preventblindness.org*
   Prevent Blindness America

August
Cataract Awareness Month   *www.eyenet.org*
   American Academy of Ophthalmology
National Immunization Awareness Month   *www.partnersforimmunization*
   National Partnership for Immunization   *.org*

August 1–7
World Breastfeeding Week   *www.lalecheleague.org*
   World Alliance for Breastfeeding Action

September
Baby Safety Month   *www.jpma.org*
   Juvenile Products Manufacturers
   Association
Cold and Flu Campaign   *www.lungusa.org*
   American Lung Association
Gynecologic Cancer Awareness Month   *www.wcn.org*
   Gynecologic Cancer Foundation
Healthy Aging Month   *www.healthyaging.net*
   Educational Television Network, Inc.
Prostate Cancer Awareness Month   *www.pcacoalition.org*
   National Prostate Cancer Coalition
Children's Eye Health and Safety Month   *www.preventblindness.org*
   Prevent Blindness America
Leukemia Awareness Month   *www.leukemia-lymphoma.org*
   Leukemia & Lymphoma Society
National Cholesterol Education Month   *www.nhlbi.nih.gov*
   National Heart, Lung, and Blood Institute
National Food Safety Education Month   *www.nraef.org/ifsc/*
   International Food Safety Council
National Lice Prevention Month   *www.headlice.org*
   National Pediculosis Association
National Sickle Cell Month   *www.sicklecelldisease.org*
   Sickle Cell Disease Association
   of America, Inc.
Ovarian Cancer Awareness Month   *www.ovarian.org*
   National Ovarian Cancer Coalition, Inc.

September 16–22
National Reye's Syndrome Week   *www.reyessyndrome.org*
   National Reye's Syndrome Foundation

September 23–30
Ulcer Awareness Week   *www.cdc.gov*
   Center for Disease Control and Prevention

October
Domestic Violence Awareness Month   *www.ncadv.org*
   National Coalition Against Domestic
   Violence
SIDS Awareness Month   *www.sidsalliance.org*
   SIDS Alliance
Family Health Month   *www.familyhealthmonth.org*
   American Academy of Family Physicians
Health Literacy Month   *www.healthliteracy.org*
   Health Literacy Counseling
Healthy Lung Month   *www.lungusa.org*
   American Lung Association
National Breast Cancer Awareness Month   *www.nbcam.org*
   National Breast Cancer Awareness Month
   Board of Sponsors
National Dental Hygiene Month   *www.adha.org*
   American Dental Hygienists' Association
National Liver Awareness Month   *www.liverfoundation.org*
   American Liver Foundation
National Lupus Awareness Month   *www.lupus.org*
   Lupus Foundation of America
National Spina Bifida Awareness Month   *www.sbaa.org*
   Spina Bifida Association of America
Rett Syndrome Awareness Month   *www.rettsyndrome.org*
   International Rett Syndrome Association

October 6–12
Mental Illness Awareness Week   *www.psych.org*
   American Psychiatric Association

October 6–12
National Fire Prevention Week   *www.nfpa.org*
   National Fire Protection Association

October 7
National Child Health Day   *www.mchb.hrsa.gov*
   U.S. Department of Health and
   Human Services

October 7–11
National School Lunch Week   *www.asfsa.org*
   American School Food Service

October 10
National Depression Screening Day   *www.mentalhealthscreening*
   National Mental Illness Screening Project   *.org*

October 13–19
National Adult Immunization   *www.nfid.org/ncai*
Awareness Week
   National Coalition for Adult
   Immunization

October 14–20
National Radon Action Week   *www.epa.gov*
   Indoor Environmental Division, EPA

October 16
World Food Day   *www.worldfooddayusa.org*
   U.S. National Committee for
   World Food Day

October 17
National Mammography Day   *www.cancer.org*
   American Cancer Society

October 21–27
National Health Education Week   *www.nche.org*
   National Center for Health Education

October 23–31
National Red Ribbon Celebration   *www.nfp.org*
   National Family Partnership

November
American Diabetes Month   *www.diabetes.org*
   American Diabetes Association
Diabetic Eye Disease Month   *www.preventblindness.org*
   Prevent Blindness America
National Alzheimer's Disease   *www.alz.org*
Awareness Month
   Alzheimer's Disease and Related
   Disorders Association
National Marrow Awareness Month   *www.marrow.org*
   National Bone Marrow Donor Program
National Epilepsy Month   *www.epilepsyfoundation.org*
   Epilepsy Foundation
National Hospice Month   *www.nhpco.org*
   National Hospice and Palliative
   Care Organization

November 17
Great American Smokeout   *www.cancer.org*
   American Cancer Society

November 24–30
GERD Awareness Week   *www.iffgd.org*
   International Foundation for Functional
   Gastrointestinal Disorders

November 18–24
National Adoption Week   *www.ncfa-usa.org*
   National Council for Adoption

December
National Drunk and Drugged   *www.3dmonth.org*
Driving (3D) Prevention Month
   3D Prevention Month Coalition
Safe Toys and Gifts Month   *www.preventblindness.org*
   Prevent Blindness America

December 1
World AIDS Day   *www.aawhworldhealth.org*
   American Association for World Health

December 1–7
National Aplastic Anemia   *www.aamds.org*
Awareness Week
   Aplastic Anemia and MDS
   International Foundation

December 8–14
National Hand Washing Awareness Week   *www.henrythehand.com*
   Henry the Hand Foundation

Keep in mind that the most important part of marketing is to make your practice stand out and create a positive, outstanding, memorable experience in the minds of your patients and potential patients.

PRESS RELEASES

The media are always looking for fresh and newsworthy stories for their audiences. A press release is a simple document that outlines your message in a certain format (Fig. 11–5). This press release, once written, can be distributed to local, state, and national media. Create a media list and enter it into your computer software so you can easily produce mailing labels. This media list should include national magazines, nursing organizations, local newspapers, television stations, radio stations, and any other media where you think your information should be published. Update this list often and try to include editors' names so the piece goes directly to the editor you wish to target. Make sure you are targeting the correct editor for your subject matter. Keep copies of the master media list handy. National and international newspaper links can

Figure 11–5 Press Release

FOR IMMEDIATE RELEASE

18 January, 1999

Contact: Carolyn Zaumeyer — (954) 776–1500

NOTE: Story has local angle

CAROLYN ZAUMEYER OF WOMEN'S HEALTH WATCH RECIEVES THE 1999 Vision In Service To Association (VISTA) AWARD

Carolyn Zaumeyer, MSN, ARNP of Ft. Lauderdale, will receive the *1999 VISTA* award by the National Association of Women Business Owners (NAWBO). The awards presentation will take place at the Westin Cypress Creek Hotel in Ft. Lauderdale on February 1, 1999. Zaumeyer has been honored as a result of her outstanding contributions to the National Association of Women Business Owners. Zaumeyer is the immediate past president and currently serves as the National Board Representative.

This year's VISTA ceremony will honor 17 "women to watch," who represent the most active and distinguished women's business organizations countywide. NAWBO is proud to have NationsBank as the Title Sponsor and expects to attract over 350 attendees.

Carolyn Zaumeyer is a graduate of Florida International University BSN, ARNP, and Master's Degree programs, having achieved Summa Cum Laude status at all three levels. Zaumeyer established an independent Nurse Practitioner gynecology practice, Women's Health Watch, over six years ago in Ft. Lauderdale. Carolyn is an author, national speaker and currently is serving as Adjunct Faculty at Florida International University.

be found at *www.webwombat.com.au/intercom/newsprs/index.htm*. If you think you need a more extensive media list, you can buy press directories:

- Publicity Blitz Media Directory on Disk, Bradley Communications at *www.rtir.com*
- All-in-One Directory, the Gebbie Press at *www.gebbieinc.com*
- Bacon's Media Catalog at *www.baconsinfo.com*

Once you have written your press release, mark off the media sources on the master list copy of which media you want to receive your press release. Modify the list for each mailing. Then, print your labels and your press release and get them in the mail in a timely fashion. You may want to include in your marketing plan scheduled press releases (monthly, quarterly, holidays).

If the story is printed, be sure to keep a nice copy of the article. Some of the articles may be worthy of a nice frame and should be hung where patients can see them. You may also want to make copies to distribute or have in your patient reception area. Seeing your name in print adds to your credibility in the patient's eyes.

The media generally responds to:

- Something "new"
- Being the first or the last
- Success—awards, recognition
- Old fashioned or futuristic themes
- Crusades for or against something
- Reversing a trend
- Funny items
- Celebrity encounters
- Breaking a record
- Human issues
- Doing the unexpected
- "est"—biggest, smallest, oldest,...
- Philanthropy
- Breaking news on health and medicine
- Helping the underserved populations
- Alternative and natural therapies
- Sex, beauty, and fitness
- Emotion

Some topics that relate specifically to your practice that the media might be interested in include:

- New practice launch
- Speaking engagements
- New services and products
- Special events
- Community activities
- Conventions or conferences
- Addition of providers to your office
- Election to board of directors of organizations
- Completion of specialized training
- Website launch
- Significant anniversaries

When producing a press release, avoid poor grammar, poor spelling, and a poor story. Do not waste your time, energy, or money putting out a less than optimal press release.

The headline and the first paragraph of copy are critical to writing a successful press release. Try to keep your press release to one page. It must be typed—never handwritten. Use double space and 1-inch margins all around. If appropriate, include one or two quotes. Keep the sentences and paragraphs short. The first paragraph should contain the "5 W's": who, what, where, when, and why. Your press release should be concise but comprehensive. Include contact information—your name, the practice's name, address, telephone, fax, and e-mail address. Traditionally this information is found on the upper left-hand corner of the press release. Use your company's letterhead or plain white paper for your press releases.

Many times, the writer will call you for more information or to clarify the information included in the press release. If you would like your information printed as soon as possible, include the statement on the upper right-hand corner of the press release "For Immediate Release." If there is a specific time when you would rather the information be printed, you can put your request in that same section, for example, "For Release on or before June 1st." The copy should be double-spaced (this gives the editor room to make notes). Be absolutely certain that every fact and title in the release is accurate and every name is spelled correctly. It is ideal to have someone read over the copy carefully to proofread for grammar, content, and spelling errors before you copy and send the press release. At the end of the copy, put the symbols ### or -30-. These symbols signify the end of the press release, signaling the reader that the release is complete. Some people think that an e-mail or fax is appropriate for a press release. If you have time constraints, you could use those methods; however, a well-written press release on quality letterhead should command more attention from the reader. Once you have designed a good press release, you can use the same format for future press releases.

PRESS INTERVIEWS

The media representatives want to have quality resources available when they need information. You should work on establishing yourself as "an expert" on health subjects. To start this process, write articles and press releases often. Published articles and books establish instant credibility. When you send articles and press releases, you can include your business card with your topics of expertise written on the back of the card. Try to develop a good relationship with the media—the results can be amazing.

According to a recent CNN/USA Today Gallup poll, second to firefighters, nurses are perceived as having the highest professional ethics and honesty. Think about this, Americans trust nurses above physicians, pharmacists, engineers, and dentists. What a great source we can be for the media.

Being interviewed by the press can be unnerving. Preparation is key for a successful interview. Prepare for interviews by deciding on a few key messages or talking points that you would like to cover during the interview. State them at the beginning, middle, and end of the interview. Try to anticipate difficult questions and other hazardous areas where the interview could lead. Practice your responses. Remember, there is no such thing as "off the record." Never say anything you wouldn't mind seeing in print. Always tell the truth. Do your research and be prepared.

The American Nurses Association is promoting a media training tool to promote nurses' expertise: *RN = Real News: "ANA Media Relations & You."* This video includes tips on media relations, specifically preparing for interviews for the radio, television, newspapers, and magazines. The video can be obtained through *www.nursebooks.org* or 1-800-637-0323.

Once you have established yourself with the media as an "expert," prepare yourself for your interview. Ask pertinent questions before you begin. For example, what is the focus of the story? When is the deadline for the story? Will the media fax or read back your quotes before they submit the article to print? What is needed for the piece—a quote, controversy, opinion, or maybe your expertise?

After the interview, be sure to send the reporter a letter thanking him or her for the opportunity. Enclose your business card along with an offer to be a source in the future. You may also want to include a copy of your curriculum vitae or resume. Also, be sure to ask when the piece will be aired or published.

TRADE SHOWS

Secure an exhibit booth at the fairs and trade shows that are attended by your target market. Decorate the exhibit space nicely. A bouquet of fresh flowers or pink roses can really soften the appearance of the traditional booth. Incorporating something with motion into your display can increase interest. Possibly using videotape on a loop that repeats or an ongoing slide show could work with either educational information or information about your practice. Think about the colors, textures, and graphics. Having a little candy or cookies for the attendees will certainly draw them to your exhibit.

Speak with the organizer of the event to optimize your exposure. Will door prizes be given away? If so, you may consider donating a door prize. Every time your practice's name is announced, the better. Be sure to bring lots of novelties with your practice's name and logo imprinted on them to give away. Consider having a drawing for a prize from your booth. This is an excellent opportunity to add to your database of "hot prospects" by collecting the attendees' names and addresses to target with mailers. Also, use this time to peruse the other exhibitors' booths for ideas for enhancing your next display. You can use this as an opportunity to network with the other exhibitors. Always be thinking about how you can work jointly with other businesses to increase your business.

To identify future trade shows contact your local school boards, travel and tourism boards, nonprofit organizations, business organizations, chambers of commerce, newspapers, colleges, universities, church groups, and even the event facilities in your area. They should have a calendar of events as well as contact and registration information available. Your local newspaper will have advertisements for upcoming events. If it is too late to participate this year, gather information so you can participate next year.

If there is a registration or booth fee, ask a few questions before committing to exhibit. Ask about past attendance, not only the total number but also the basic demographics of attendees if available. Is this your target market? Should you be spending your time, money, and energy on this group? Ask how many booths they plan to sell—the more, the better. Are there any other exhibitors from your practice specialty? Can you promote the event to your patient base to increase attendance?

NEWSLETTERS/E-ZINES

Publishing a newsletter for your current and prospective patients is a great way to promote your practice. Newsletters help keep your name in front of your patients and prospective patients. It doesn't necessarily need to be weekly or even monthly. A quarterly newsletter could include information on your speaking and research activities. You could include health tips and health information. A coupon for specific specials could be included as well. This newsletter could be handed out at networking and speaking functions to promote your practice. It could be mailed to prospective patients. This newsletter does not have to be expensive—you can design it on your computer, print out a clear copy, and have it printed at an office supply store.

Newsletters should be designed to show your patients that you care about them and their health. You can use the newsletter to reinforce the health-care messages that you would like to convey to your patients. You will appear as the caring expert; this may contribute to your credibility in the community. The newsletter can make your practice look even bigger and more professional while still conveying warmth and concern.

When planning your newsletter, first think about your goal or purpose of the newsletter. To whom are you targeting the newsletter? Is it more for marketing or education? Or maybe the newsletter will be a combination of both? How often do you plan on publishing your newsletter?

What size newsletter do you feel would be best for your target market? One to four pages is the norm. What is your budget? Whether you can afford to produce the newsletter and mail it to all of your current and prospective patients, or if you are producing it for a handout—a professional printer will print a newsletter to be proud of. Handing out a poorly printed piece from your office copier will not be presenting your business in the most professional light. Your newsletter is an extension of you and your practice. Be sure it conveys the image that you want your patients to remember.

E-zines are newsletters sent via the Internet to e-mail addresses. If you have collected e-mail addresses for your target audience, this can be a very effective and inexpensive way to promote your practice. To create an e-zine, you need an e-mail account and permission from your patients to send the e-zine. When collecting the e-mail addresses, you may want to tell the patients of some of the benefits to receiving an e-zine from your practice. Some of the benefits may include up-to-date health care information, special offers, discounts, and contests. Be sure to list your services and products in all of your newsletters and e-zines.

When designing your e-zine, keep it simple. Make it a quick and easy read. Usually two to three pages is enough room to let the reader know you are thinking of them and to share news. If you are interested in investigating e-zines, there is a great software program that you purchase once (no monthly fee) that you may want to investigate. To investigate this software program, visit *http://www.SellShareware.com/ProgramInfo.asp?AfID=7838&PrID=34362.*

If you have developed a Website for your practice, add a subscription area for your e-zine. You may want to include on your patient information sheet a space for the patient to write in his or her e-mail address so you can start your e-mail database. You could also have a sign-up sheet in the reception area outlining what the e-zine includes (maybe attach a sample e-zine). Tell anyone you think may have an interest in receiving your newsletter. At networking functions and trade shows, you may want to have a sign-up sheet out with a sample if it is appropriate.

COMMUNITY INVOLVEMENT

Depending on your target market, you may want to volunteer to speak at high schools or adult centers. Maximize your efforts with good publicity by sending out press releases. Make yourself available to speak at career-days at the local schools. Volunteering your time at local community and health centers can lead to increased exposure to yourself and your practice. The more contact you have with potential referral sites, the better.

Donate gift certificates or a gift basket of your products to charity events. Sponsor or host a charity or business marketing event at your office (if space permits). The more people who see how nice and professional your office is, the better. You could even host an educational meeting for the public at your office and you could speak on health topics that relate to your practice.

Many churches and synagogues have scheduled educational programs and seminars. Many times they are looking for good speakers. You may want to put together a promotional package introducing yourself, your practice, speaking history, and availability to speak. Within the packet, include a listing of topics that you are prepared to speak about. The more exposure, the better!

Some local organizations sponsor health fairs and are looking for exhibitors. This is an inexpensive way to distribute your promotional materials. Take care when designing your display area. Make it educational, professional, but also approachable. If you have set up a booth or display, it is much more effective if you or your employees are there to answer questions and generate interest. You should be visible and active in your professional community and with the lay communities as much as possible.

You could donate your time for specialty consultation or hold educational programs on specific health concerns. Some areas you may want to explore include smoking cessation, child safety, teaching breast self-exam, weight loss, health, fitness, skin care, anxiety, depression, and sexual health issues. The word of mouth advertisements you receive from these donations of your time and knowledge are certain to pay off in the long run.

GRAND OPENING

This can be a very exciting time in your business development. Things are coming together and are about to take off. Starting off on the right foot can lead to great times ahead. The importance of getting the word out to the community that you are starting your own practice is of the utmost importance. People need to know that you have opened your practice and are ready for business.

Before hanging the "Grand Opening" or "Open for Business," signs you should double check all of the systems in place that will guarantee that your first days of patient care will be successful. One of the best exercises that will test the readiness of your office, staff, and yourself is to do a mock patient encounter. Have a friend or family member arrive through the front door as if he or she were your first patient. Have your staff prepared to great and process this person as if he or she were the first to come through the door. Monitor their wording, sincerity, and completeness of required activities. Have the staff prepare a chart and bring the "patient" to the appropriate area (lab, your office, or exam room) for the visit.

Once the staff is done and the patient is waiting for you, it is your turn to make sure you are ready. Take the patient through your full exam (but with clothes on!). Make sure you have all of the supplies and equipment you need to complete the exam. Once you are done and have written the appropriate prescriptions and marked your superbill with the appropriate billing codes, bring the patient up to the front desk to check out. Have the front office staff go through the entire process of checking out the patient.

After your mock exam is done, sit down and have a discussion with everyone involved—including your "patient." Get feedback from them all and let them help each other to refine their processes. In the first few months of business, you will all be learning and changing your activities. It is good to establish an open discussion and get your "team" working together to make your patients' visits as pleasant, comfortable, and efficient as possible.

Your grand opening celebration is not just a party to launch your new practice; it is a great time to market your practice. To do it right, you should send out printed invitations for the event (Fig. 11–6).

Your mailing list should be comprised of people who have the power to help you grow your practice, such as your banker, accountant, friends, family, neighbors, any professionals who can refer business to you, and any other people who have helped you start the practice. If you have a large database of people to whom you would like to announce the starting of your practice, but whom you do not necessarily want to invite to the grand opening, you can print up a nice announcement. Be sure to include your business card in the mailings.

Figure 11–6   Sample Open House Invitation

Open House Celebration!
You are invited to help us
commemorate the official
grand opening of our new

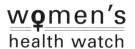

women's
health watch

A Progressive Health Care Center
For Today's Woman

Carolyn Zaumeyer, MSN, ARNP

Date: Friday, January 14, 20_ _
Time: 4:00 p.m. to 7:00 p.m.
Place: 1234 North Westend St.
Goodtown, USA 56789
(123) 456-7890

Informal

You can purchase an inexpensive "Grand Opening" sign to hang outside your practice for the first month for added recognition.

The actual party can be simple hors d'oeuvres (either purchased or home made), soda, and maybe beer and wine. Be sure to have plenty of plates, cups, napkins, ice, and supplies. Have your office absolutely sparkling clean and looking its best.

Have your brochure, flyers, business cards, and any other promotional material displayed. Remember, the more printed material handed out, the better.

A well-written press release with a photo of yourself should be mailed to the local papers and nursing newsletters. Relax and enjoy the moment. Just think, how many times in your life will you be starting your own practice?

MAINTAINING YOUR PATIENT BASE

When looking at your marketing budget, you will see that it costs a lot of money to get new patients established in your practice. It doesn't cost anything to get current patients to spend more. What it costs is your time in identifying what collateral services or products are appropriate and then offering the service or product to your patients. Your patients know you and trust you, and are likely to take your advice. As long as your advice is appropriate, there is nothing wrong with offering extra services and products. You may ask yourself "Am I selling a service or product the patient doesn't want?" Many times patients will thank you for offering extra services or products—just don't push. You can even train your staff to suggest potential services or products. Be sure to offer services and products that your patient want and need.

Display a listing of services and products offered at your office in the reception area. The last thing you want to hear from a long-time patient is "I didn't know you did that! I could have been coming to you for that service all of these years!" A simple sign posted in the reception area outlining any specials you have put together can help increase your revenues.

Contact patients who have not been in your office in the past 12 months with either a friendly telephone call or a postcard. When you add a new service or product, let your patients know. Post it in the reception area and then tell them about it.

Sending a birthday card to your established patients is very much appreciated. You may even consider inserting a lotto card ($1) for that week. This little gesture goes far. The patients are surprised and they tell their friends and family members. This simple act generates great "word of mouth" advertising.

Devise a system for thanking your patients for referring new patients. You may want to create a "Send a Friend" referral program wherein the referring patient is rewarded with a discount or a gift certificate. Let your patients know that you need and appreciate all referrals.

Returning phone calls promptly will go a long way with your patients. If you think of a patient and wonder how he or she is doing, then call. Chances are the patient will be so pleased that you have called that he or she will tell other people about it. What great free advertising!

Take the time to listen to your patient. Not only will the patient help direct you to the diagnosis quicker than by your just examining the patient, but this makes the patient feel good about your interaction. Rushing through your patient encounter can undo all of the good marketing you have done. Patients want you to be focused on them and spend as much time as necessary to meet their needs. However, you must also be respectful of their time. If they are seeing you during their lunch hour for a simple visit, do your best to get them back to work on time while still providing the services that they expect and deserve. A good policy is to keep the patient waiting no longer than 15 minutes before being seen by you. This is very possible with good scheduling and is truly appreciated by the patients. Have you ever been kept waiting for 45 minutes or more to see a health-care provider? It doesn't feel good.

Everyone likes the feeling of *being important*. Let your patients know how important they are to you. Let your staff know how important it is that your patients are to be considered very important. You may want to take a few minutes and create a statement about the importance of your patients. Your statement may include thoughts such as: "Our patients come first, no one is more important than our patients, our patients are not an interruption of our work—they are the purpose of our work." Once you have fine-tuned your statement, print it up nicely, frame it and then hang it in your employees' work area. It is good to have a reminder for your employees; also, the patients will enjoy seeing your philosophy on your patient relations. As a consumer, you know how you want to be treated and you know how you don't want to be treated. It is much less expensive to build onto your current patient base rather than to constantly replace your patient base.

Discuss with your staff how you would like them to handle patient complaints. Hopefully this won't be an issue to deal with often, but if handled correctly, you will be able to satisfy the patient as well as keeping your office running smoothly. One approach is to direct any controversies to one specific staff member (office manager or yourself) to resolve the issue. Strive to resolve the issue without creating a major commotion in front of other patients. If there are others around, you may want to take the patient to a private area to discuss the complaint. This is a time to employ those listening skills you have been working on. Let the patient talk and vent as long as possible. He or she may feel better once the concerns have been heard. Some people love to complain and push other people around. Handle these people with care. Most malpractice suits come from patients who believe that they were not treated nicely or with respect from the provider and their staff. Empathize with the patient, stay calm, and take responsibility.

There is a wonderful resource that could be helpful with patient satisfaction: *Managing Patient Expectations: The Art of Finding and Keeping Loyal Patients* by Susan Keane Baker. Patients may not only be looking for a healthcare provider, but also for a relationship and possibly a friendship.

On a regular basis you should assess your current versus previous patient list. If a patient hasn't been into the office within a certain amount of time, say 1 year, you may need to send a reminder that you are still in business and you miss the patient. This can be a simple telephone call or an inexpensive postcard. On the postcard, you may want to offer a discount or something for free at the patient's next visit. If you include a coupon on the postcard, you will be able to track the success of your mailing project. Include an expiration date on the coupon to encourage the patient to schedule soon. Be sure to update your database with address changes and returned cards so you don't waste future marketing money on incorrect addresses.

Listen to your patients, identify their needs, take care of those needs, and fulfill their expectations. Feel free to ask patients why they come to you and not the competition. You may be surprised by their answers. Write their responses down in a log. Their comments may help you when promoting your practice. Some people may be so bold during networking to ask you "why should I come to you instead of my regular doctor?" You can be prepared for such questions by using the comments of your current patients. Also, ask former patients why they are not using your services any longer. You can learn a lot by asking questions. Remember, if you don't take care of your patients, someone else will.

COMMENT CARD/PATIENT SATISFACTION SURVEY

It is nice to learn what you are doing well with your practice. However, it may be more valuable to learn what you could be doing better. Comment cards are a simple and inexpensive way to fine-tune the operations of your practice. Take some time to think through what you really want to learn from your patients.

Limit your questionnaire to one page with no more than 12 questions with check-off answers. You can allow for one open-ended question area for "Any additional comments or suggestions." Make it easy to complete and return. You may ask patients to complete the questionnaire before they leave as their charges are being processed. If you send the questionnaire by mail, be sure to include a stamped card or envelope, your fax number, and address. You may want to create some type of a monthly or quarterly drawing for those that complete the survey. A simple $5 off their next visit may inspire your patients to take the time to complete the survey. Share or post the results of your survey. People like to know how others feel about your practice.

Some areas you may want to ask about include:

- Courtesy of office staff
- Ease of scheduling appointment
- Cleanliness of office
- Quality of service
- Services provided
- Price of services
- Office location
- Billing procedures
- Hours of service
- Parking area

The above areas could be ranked with a check-off system using "excellent," "good," "fair," and "poor." You could also ask if they would be willing to use your services again and if they would be willing to recommend your practice to others. A simple "yes," "no," and "not sure" check-off area would work well for these questions. Be sure to thank the patients for their time and thoughts (Fig. 11–7).

NOVELTIES

Advertising specialty items or novelties are usually inexpensive items that keep your name in front of current and future patients. These items are helpful in promoting your practice. Even though they may be inexpensive, people do enjoy receiving free things! You can give them to patients and also distribute them at networking and trade show events. There are many to choose from, such as calendars, mouse pads, notepads, pens, pencils, emery boards, mugs, refrigerator magnets, customized book marks, water bottles, stress balls, stuffed animals, key chains, rulers, balloons, and letter openers.

When deciding which advertising novelties to order, evaluate a few things:

- What is the cost per item?
- Where and how will you distribute these items?
- Does the item fit in with your practice specialty or slogan?
- Will your logo or practice information fit on the item?
- Does the item's quality and style reflect the image you want to project?

There are many sources for purchasing your novelties; be sure to see samples and proofread the artwork before the final order is placed. You don't want to receive 1,000 calendars with your practice name spelled incorrectly! Chic Ideas, Inc., has a unique collection of high-quality items. These items can be viewed and purchased at *www.chicideas.com*.

| **Figure 11–7** | **Sample Patient Satisfaction Survey** |

Insert your logo, address and phone here

HOW ARE WE DOING?

Because your satisfaction is the key to our success, we are always interested in improving our services to you. We strive to be the best in our field, and your information is crucial to helping us maintain the finest quality of service. Thank you for taking a moment to let us know how we are doing.

Please rate the following:

	Excellent	Good	Fair	Poor
1. Services provided	☐	☐	☐	☐
2. Courtesy of staff	☐	☐	☐	☐
3. Office cleanliness	☐	☐	☐	☐
4. Quality of service	☐	☐	☐	☐
5. Price of service	☐	☐	☐	☐
6. Speed of service	☐	☐	☐	☐
7. Office location	☐	☐	☐	☐
8. Billing procedures	☐	☐	☐	☐
9. Hours of service	☐	☐	☐	☐
10. Ease of appointment	☐	☐	☐	☐

	Yes	No	Not Sure
11. Would you be willing to use our services again?	☐	☐	☐
12. Would you be willing to recommend our services?	☐	☐	☐

13. Any additional comments or suggestions?

_____

_____

Thank you for your time and information. We hope we can serve you again soon.

CONTESTS

A fun way to increase your publicity and patient loyalty is to host a contest. You can do this along with other businesses or just on your own. You may want to do a monthly, quarterly, or annual contest, or possibly link it to a holiday that works with your specialty (e.g., cardiac—Valentines Day; occupational medicine—Labor Day). You can even link up with the nontraditional holidays. You can purchase a calendar with all the traditional and nontraditional recognition days and holidays at *www.chases.com.*

Your contest can be a simple drawing (this is good to do at trade shows too). Have the patients or prospective patients write their name, address, and telephone number on a piece of paper, drop it into a bowl, and you have a contest! You can also increase your database for future marketing projects. You can certainly be more elaborate with different submission requirements (e.g., coloring for pediatrics, guessing games, trivia.).

The prize for your contest is totally up to you. You want to make it appealing so you have maximum participation and people talk about it. Try to tie the prize into promoting your practice while rewarding the participant. If it is a unique or remarkable prize, be sure to maximize your publicity with a well-written press release. Be sure to publicize your contest by handing out flyers and telling everyone about the contest.

Another option is to sponsor and promote a contest or sweepstakes and have the beneficiary be a local charity. You could even partner with the charity to maximize the publicity. By teaming with a charity, you may be able to get a lot more free press and free advertising.

MONITORING YOUR MARKETING EFFORTS

All of your marketing efforts and expenditures need to be examined and evaluated on a regular basis. The key question you need to answer is "How are my new patients learning about my practice?" As you know, if you don't have patients, you don't have a practice. Whether you have the patients write on their initial patient information sheet where they first learned of your practice or you keep a sheet next to the telephone and log where the callers learned of the practice—this is a very important activity.

Ascertaining how your patients first heard of your practice will help with future marketing planning and spending. If your computer software can track this information, it should be easy to compile your data on a regular basis. If you get more than 50% of your patients from the yellow pages, your listing is very effective and must be continued. It is also important to know what marketing venues are not effective. Then, you can direct your marketing time, effort, and money in the best areas possible.

SCRAPBOOK

It may sound a little juvenile to suggest starting a scrapbook. However, a scrapbook can assist you when you review your marketing efforts as well as review your career achievements. A simple scrapbook from Hallmark can give you a nice cover and heavy pages to attach your advertisements, grand opening invitation, announcements, photos, articles, and anything else you would like to remember.

Some people create a "marketing only" scrapbook. Inside they put a copy of their advertisements, how much they cost, where it was run, dates, and for how long. Also, if possible, write in the response to the advertisement. If you are using different coupons with each marketing endeavor, you can note the number of coupons redeemed. This can give you concrete information to evaluate your current and future marketing efforts, time, and money.

COMMON MARKETING MISTAKES

Learning as you go is very important. Pay attention to your marketing efforts. Some of the most common marketing mistakes include:

- Failure to plan your marketing strategy
- Failure to follow your marketing plan
- Failure to advertise
- Failure to distinguish the difference between you and your competitors
- Pitching to the wrong markets
- Failure to take advantage of the press
- Failure to remain involved in your practice's marketing efforts
- Failure to share services and products available
- Failure to highlight one's medical specialty
- Failure to encourage word of mouth
- Failure to develop, maintain, and use a marketing database
- Failure to network

You have now been given the tools to create and implement a good marketing plan. This is definitely an area that warrants constant attention. This is a fun and interesting area of your practice that was probably not addressed during your nurse's training. However, with a little bit of work and perseverance, you can become proficient at marketing your practice.

SUGGESTIONS AND TIPS FROM WOMEN'S HEALTH WATCH, INC.

■ During the first month of business, I began marketing Women's Health Watch at the local meetings of NAWBO (National Association of Women Business Owners). Through networking efforts with this organization, Women's Health Watch had exposure to hundreds of women. These women not only became patients but also became friends, colleagues, and advisors. The wealth of knowledge and experience of these women is mind-blowing. I was able to grow my business with new relationships with bankers, accountants, marketing experts, telephone company executives, and much more.

■ The comment card we used at Women's Health Watch gave us very valuable information. We tallied the results monthly and actually produced reports rating our different areas surveyed.

■ When evaluating your marketing efforts, realize it may take time to reap the benefits of your advertising. Patients would sometimes carry in a copy of an advertisement from the grand opening announcement in the newspaper 2 or 3 years after we opened!

PERSONAL ANECDOTES

1. I became known among my friends and colleagues as the "Press Release Queen." Whenever the opportunity arises to send out a press release, I do. I also include a photograph of myself whenever it is appropriate. My friends have admitted that the reason they tease me is that they are envious of all the press my practice and I receive! It could be you and your new practice receiving free exposure if you do your homework.

2. Many new business owners think that the cost of creating a logo for their new business is an unnecessary expense. My logo has raised many comments and has become more recognizable than my name could ever have become without the logo. I get compliments on my business cards when I hand them out. I feel comfortable that they represent the quality and image my practice should project.

3. If you have a unique hobby or other activity that may attract the press, be sure to mention your practice if you are interviewed. A local female CPA rides a motorcycle and is interviewed often. She always says her name is Laura Weiner, CPA. She has become a celebrity of sorts and is recognized as being a CPA too. So, tie your hobby into your business if you can for extra exposure.

4. Look for a unique educational tool you can develop to promote your practice. A female body shop owner created a handy little brochure on "What to do if you are in an accident." It was a simple design that outlined step-by-step the actions you should take if you are in an auto accident. The best part was that she included her company name and telephone number at the bottom of the brochure in large bold print. People would keep this information in their glove compartments and refer to it during their time of need. Then, they could simply call her shop to make arrangements for the repairs to their automobile—how clever!

5. You may not enjoy marketing your practice in the beginning. It may be uncomfortable for you to be presenting yourself to the community. However, it is part of the role of being a business owner. You must promote your practice or you may end up without a practice to promote. It is easy to get wrapped up in the day-to-day activities of running a practice. Marketing the practice should be included in your day-to-day duties. Don't drop the ball.

Resources

2001 Media Guide to Health Care Experts. Sigma Theta Tau International: *www.nursingsociety.org.*

All-in-One Directory. Gebbie Press, Inc: *www.gebbieinc.com.*

American Academy of Nurse Practitioners: Nurse practitioner brochures and videotape: *www.aanp.org.*

Bacon's Media Catalog: *www.baconsinfo.com.*

Booher, D. To the letter: A handbook of model letters for the busy manager. New York, Lexington Books, 1998.

Calendars: Traditional and non-traditional recognition days: *www.chases.com.*

Ccnow: Internet credit card processing: *www.ccnow.com.*

Chic Ideas, Inc: Novelties: *www.chicideas.com* or 954-587-5316.

Frisk-E-Business: Free Marketing e-zine, subscribe at *Heidi@FriskEBusiness.com.*

Hiam, A: Marketing for dummies. NY, Hungry Minds, 1997.

ImageCafe: Web page design: *www.imagecafe.com.*

Keane Baker, S: Managing patient expectations: The art of finding and keeping loyal patients. San Francisco, Jossey-Bass, 1998.

Leduc, B: How to build your small business fast with simple post cards: *www.BobLeduc.com,* 2000.

Media Networks: Major advertising opportunities: *www.medianetworks.com.*

McIntyre, CV: Writing effective news releases…: How to get free publicity for yourself, your business or your organization. Colorado Springs, Piccadilly Books, 1992.

Michaels, N., and Karpowicz, DJ: Off the wall marketing ideas: Jumpstart your sales without busting your budget. Holbrook, MA, Adams Media, 2000.

Miller, SK: Marketing your practice. Patient Care for the Nurse Practitioner 11:52–53, 2000.

Newspaper links: *www.webwombat.com.au/intercom/newsprs/index.htm.*

NP Central: Brochures, directory sample letter and registry at *www.nurse.net.*

NP Clinics: Registry: *www.npclinics.com*.

Nurses rank no. 2 in Gallup "honesty and ethics" poll: The American Nurse 2(5), 2002.

Parkhurst, W: How to get publicity and make the most of it once you've got it. San Francisco, Harpers Business, 2000.

Plan Magic Marketing 6.0 [computer software]: Jefferson, Valley, NY, PlanMagic Corporation, 2001: *www.planmagic.com*.

PlanWrite for Marketing [computer software]: Austin, TX, Business Resource Software, 2001: *www.brs-inc.com*.

Publicity Blitz Media Directory: *www.rtir.com*.

Richards, H: Rose marketing on a daisy budget. Miramar, FL, WUN Publications, 1999.

RN = Real News: ANA Media Relations & You. American Nurses Association, 2000: *www.nursebooks.org*.

Rosen, E: The anatomy of buzz: How to create word-of-mouth marketing. New York, Doubleday, 2000.

Sell Shareware: E-zine software program: *www.SellShareware.com/ProgramInfo.asp?AfID=7838&PrID=34362*.

Small Business Association: *www.sba.gov*.

Smithing, RT: Nurse practitioners: A secret no more. Nurse Practitioner World News 9:3–10, 2001.

VeriSign: Domain name registration: *www.netsol.com*.

Wilson, JR: Word-of-mouth marketing. Fort Worth, TX, Branch-Smith Publications, 2000.

N O T E S

Chapter 12

Managing the Finances: How Do I Do It?

" Beware of little expenses, a small leak will sink a great ship "

Benjamin Franklin

Keeping the books properly is critical to business success and profitability. Accurate records are essential for planning and making informed management decisions. Some other reasons to maintain precise records are to track interactions with others, supply present and potential lenders with correct financial data, comply with government regulations, detail taxable income, and provide information on the growth of your business.

There are many resources available to assist you with handling the financial aspects of your practice. One of the most complete and helpful resources is a cross-governmental collaborative project produced by the Small Business Administration (SBA) along with the Internal Revenue Service (IRS)—*The Small Business Resource Guide CD-ROM*. This is available at no cost either by calling 1-800-829-3676 or by visiting the IRS Website at *http://www.irs.gov.* The *Small Business Resource Guide* provides all of the IRS tax forms, instructions, and publications needed by small business owners. It also includes information on writing a business plan, finding financing for your business, and much more. The publication *Starting a Business and Keeping Records* may also be helpful. This publication can be downloaded from *http://www.irs.gov.*

SETTING UP YOUR ACCOUNTING SYSTEM

If you haven't hired an accountant, now is the time. Collaborating with an accountant now will help you avoid wasting both time and money in the future. Since all of our practices are a bit different, so are our accounting needs.

Accounting software can streamline your bookkeeping processes. By using the software, you can save time as well as produce financial reports that may help your business grow.

QuickBooks Pro by Intuit (*Quicken.com* or 1-888-2-Intuit) is a very good and reliable program. This program can help you with keeping bank records, payroll taxes, and financial reports. It is easy to use and a worthwhile investment. You will input information about your bank accounts, credit cards, debt, and payroll. You can even write checks and print them on your computer printer. Your accountant can help you set up your "chart of accounts" in a way that will make your tax preparation process much easier. The chart of accounts serves as an index to your business regarding deposits and checks written. A number is assigned to the account and helps organize your bookkeeping. At the end of the year, you can simply hand your accountant a copy of your accounts on a disk (or attach the file to an e-mail) that contains most of the information needed to complete your annual tax forms.

When designing your practice, you should make it very clear which responsibilities are yours, which are your staff's, and which are the certified public accountant's (CPA's). You may want to sit with your accountant and your staff to go over the bookkeeping duties and make assignments (Fig. 12–1). Your CPA should be available to answer questions so you can start off on the right foot. You want to know who is doing what and when. You must keep your finger on the pulse of your business—or else it may expire!

INTERVIEWING AND HIRING A CPA

The best way to find a CPA is to ask around. Ask other people with medical practices or small businesses who they use as their CPA. And, most importantly, are they happy with the services provided? You can also look in the Yellow Pages under "Accountants, CPA."

When first calling a CPA, explain that you are starting a small business and that you are looking for an accountant who handles primarily small business clients. Once this is established, briefly describe your business. Don't immediately inquire about fees. First ask the CPA how your account would be handled. This gives you the opportunity to hear him or her speak. Listen for any of the following things during the conversation:

- A good CPA would be interested in what kind of an entity you will be using to operate your business (e.g., sole proprietorship, corporation, partnership, or limited liability company). The CPA should want to help you decide which entity is best in your particular situation.
- The CPA should then want to discuss whether you'll be liable for payroll taxes, sales taxes, and any other taxes particular to the state

Figure 12-1	Bookkeeping Assignment Sheet

Task	CPA	You	Staff #1 name _____	Staff #2 name _____	When
Write checks/ pay bills					
Sign checks					
Prepare deposit slips					
Take deposits to bank					
Open mail					
Reconcile bank statements					
Communicate with CPA					
Obtain necessary tax forms					
Complete and file tax forms:					
Quarterly 941					
Annual 1120					
State taxes					
Print monthly financial reports					
Open insurance payments and post to accounts					
Collect and organize tax deductible receipts					
Organize, then forward records for annual tax returns to CPA					
Payroll					

and city in which you live. You will want a CPA who will educate you on these taxes and help you file the required paperwork on time! A responsible CPA will put your information in a database so as not to miss any filing deadlines.

■ Next, you'll want to discuss what method of bookkeeping you'll use, whether you'll be entering your expenses into a computerized accounting program yourself or sending your bank statements and check stubs to the CPA to enter.

■ Finally, you'll want to hear which expenses are deductible in your particular business and how to properly account for the business portions of your automobile usage and entertainment.

■ When you find a CPA you would consider retaining, ask about fees. This way, you can hear what services you'll be getting for the fees the CPA will be charging. If for some reason, you don't feel comfortable with this CPA, interview a couple more until you find one you like. You must be able to have good, open conversations with your CPA. And, don't let the CPA intimidate you with language you don't understand! If you don't understand something, speak up! Be sure to take good notes during the interview so there are no misunderstandings later.

You must work *with* your CPA by giving him or her all of the documentation needed to support every deduction on your return. Just as you expect your patients to follow your plan, you have the responsibility of helping your CPA understand your tax-related documents. By organizing your documents, you will save money; if you don't, you will be paying a high rate for them to sort through your receipts to try to make sense of them.

Your CPA will be your advocate in the financial world. Your CPA can help you with tax planning. He or she can let you know exactly what you can and cannot deduct from your taxes. Just as we appreciate patients who take the time to learn about their health, your CPA appreciates clients who take the time to learn about their finances.

BANKING

You should shop for your bank just as you shop for your medical supplies. Gather information on what they can and will do for you. Find out what the different "small business banking" programs have to offer. Investigate and compare the monthly service charges. Check out how much the bank charges for printing checks and deposit slips. Must you maintain a minimum balance in your checking account? Will you earn interest if you keep a high balance? Is there a program to cover checking overdrafts from your savings account? Will you receive a credit card or line of credit for your business? What is the charge if a patient writes a bad check? Is there a delay when deposits are made from out of state? Can you drop off night deposits? What online banking services are available? Will you have a personal bank representative with whom you can develop a relationship and call with questions?

All of your bank accounts should be reconciled every month when the statements arrive. Unless you are writing the checks and reconciling your accounts yourself, someone other than the person writing the checks must do the monthly bank reconciliation. Be very careful when you are assigning duties that have to do with your business' money—don't set yourself up to be robbed. Keep your checks locked up and never leave signed blank checks around. Be sure to print and save all copies of reconciliation reports that you generate. You may want to have the bank statements mailed to your home address so you can see what checks are going through your account. It is just another way to help you prevent and identify fraud. Remember, someone who may have gained your trust may be tempted to embezzle your practice's funds. Be careful.

FINANCIAL STATEMENTS

We didn't learn accounting terminology in nursing school, but it isn't too late. You may be gaining most of your business knowledge now as you develop your business. That is okay. At least you are taking the time to learn it now.

Monthly financial statements are easily prepared with your accounting software program. You should print out relevant reports monthly for comparison. You can track your growth and maybe identify areas of concern. Some of the reports you may want to print out and review include income statements, cash flow statements, and balance sheets. Lenders ask for these specific reports.

The income statement demonstrates the ability of your business to generate revenue. The income statement considers account revenue, cost of goods sold, gross profit, and other factors. This should be reviewed monthly, especially during your first year of business. The cash flow statement can be one of the most useful tools in managing your business. This spreadsheet monitors the health of your business. It starts with the cash on hand and sources of income, and deducts expenses and capital requirements, thereby producing net cash flow. This figure is carried over to the next month as the beginning cash.

The balance sheet is generally produced on an annual basis. It summarizes all financial information into assets, liabilities, and equity. This is usually required when you are applying for financing. Balance sheets are used to calculate the net worth of the business.

With these reports you should be able to estimate what your monthly overhead usually costs the business. You need to know approximately how much income you need to cover your expenses. For example, if your overhead runs around $10,000 per month you need to bring in approximately $2,500 per week. If you are short one week, you may want to encourage more laboratory screening or other revenue-producing products or services. It may feel strange to think about patient care in terms of dollars; however, you are now running a business. Without income, you cannot continue to provide quality health care to your community.

PAYROLL TAXES

You are going to learn more about taxes than you ever wanted to know! You will also pay more taxes than you ever imagined possible! It is very important that you learn the tax laws and follow them. Federal and state income taxes are some of the most significant costs a business faces. The Internal Revenue Service and most states require employers to make appropriate withholdings from employee wages. Failure to comply with the laws can lead to penalties and interest as well as liens against the owner's property. Employers are required to withhold from their employee's payroll the following:

- Federal income tax
- State income tax (in most states)
- Federal Insurance Contributions Act (FICA—Social Security)
- Worker's compensation (in some states)

There are numerous report forms and filing requirements. Your CPA can give you guidance so you comply with all of the laws. An annual earnings statement must be prepared for each employee at the end of the calendar year. It is required that the Social Security Administration and the state/city/local departments of revenue receive W-2 forms by the last day in February. Employees must receive complete W-2 Wage and Tax statements by January 31 each year. The Employer's Tax Guide Circular E contains withholding tables, Social Security, and federal unemployment information.

You must have a taxpayer identification number or employer identification number (EIN) so the IRS can process your returns. You must fill out an application Form SS-4, *Application for Employer Identification Number.* You can get Form SS-4 at Social Security Administration offices or by calling the IRS at 1-800-829-3676. If you apply by telephone, you can get an EIN immediately. Through the mail it may take 4 to 5 weeks to receive your EIN. More information on the EIN is available at *http://www.irs.gov.*

Employer's Quarterly Federal (payroll) Tax Return (Form 941) and Deposit Coupons (Form 8109) are forms you will come to know quite well. Form 941 is filed 1 month after the end of each calendar quarter with the IRS regional office. This form reports FICA and withheld income taxes on wages. Circular E provides tax tables that determine the individual employee's withholding amount. You will generally deposit taxes withheld under either a monthly or semi-weekly rule. Deposits must be made with the correct deposit coupons. You will receive deposit coupons from the IRS at the start of each new payroll quarter.

You may file Form 941 over the Internet. By filing Form 941 electronically, returns are processed quickly and calculation errors are virtually eliminated. Tight electronic security ensures confidentiality of the data. To use this service, employers must first submit an application, which is found at *http://www.nationtax.com.* More information about filing Form 941 and other federal business taxes is available on the IRS Website at *http://www.irs.gov/ elec_svc/efile-bus.html,* or by calling 1-877-786-3453.

There are payroll services available that will (for a nominal charge) write the payroll checks and figure the deductions. Two national payroll services are Paychex at *www.paychex.com* or 1-800-322-7292 and ADP (Automatic Data Processing) at *www.adp.com* or 1-800-225-5237. They also provide other human resource services, such as providing employee handbooks, 401K services, and direct deposit.

SALES TAX

If you sell products such as vitamins, health products, and books from your practice, then you should consult your CPA regarding potential state sales tax applicable to those products. If your state requires you to collect sales tax on products, learn the percentage required and then add that on to the cost to the patient. Set up a sales log system to record all taxable sales. This makes filing your tax forms much easier.

OTHER TAXES

You may be required to pay additional taxes. If you own property, you will probably have to pay taxes on the property. If you own your building and rent it to your practice, you may have to pay state sales tax on the rent. Many states require intangible and tangible state tax payments. Your CPA will be able to guide you on all of your tax requirements.

TAX DEDUCTIONS

Make a list of all of the items you think should be tax deductible—for example, attorneys fees, accountant fees, office expenses, car expenses, gifts, charitable donations, travel, cellular telephone, office equipment, membership dues, books, educational materials, lab coats, and so on. Ask your CPA about each item and write down the answer given. Ask your CPA if he or she can think of anything else you should be aware of regarding deductions. Ask what documentation is needed for each item to be considered a deduction. Set up a filing system to keep these documents in order. It is also a good idea to keep a calendar up-to-date on required tax filing for your practice.

SUGGESTIONS AND TIPS FROM WOMEN'S HEALTH WATCH, INC.

- Make friends with your money—take a "hands on" role with accountants and bankers. Learn as you go. Don't just say "Okay" if you don't really understand what they are saying. No one cares about your money more than you do!
- Join support and networking groups. Many groups have educational meetings that will contain valuable information for your business.

PERSONAL ANECDOTE

I met my CPA at a local meeting of the National Association of Women Business Owners. We started working together planning a large awards banquet. From our committee work together, I got to know her and I knew we would be able to have a good working relationship together. My relationship with my CPA has been fantastic. I have learned so much from her. It gives me a great sense of security knowing my practice's finances are in capable hands.

Resources

ADP (Automatic Data Processing): *www.adp.com* or 1-800-225-5237.

Chang, CF, et al: Economics and Nursing: Critical Professional Issues. FA Davis, Philadelphia, 2001.

Employer Identification Number information: *http://www.irs.gov/forms_pubs/pubs/p58303.htm*.

IRS electronic filing information: *http://www.irs.gov/elec_svc/efile-bus.html* or 512-460-8900.

Mancuso, JR: Mancuso's Small Business Resource Guide, 2nd ed. Small Business Source Books, New York, 1996.

Murray, D: Prepare to meet your preparer. Medical Economics Magazine [online, February 8, 1999], 20: *http://www.pdr.net/memag/static.htm?path=docs/020899/article1.html*.

Nationtax Online (Form 941 electronic filing): *http://www.nationtax.com* or 1-877-786-3453.

Paychex: *www.paychex.com* or 1-800-322-7292.

QuickBooks or QuickBooks Pro by Intuit: *www.quicken.com* or 1-888-2-Intuit.

The Small Business Resource Guide CD-ROM: *http://www.irs.gov/bus_info/sm_bus/smbus-cd.html* or 1-800-829-3676.

NOTES

Chapter 13

Managing Your Employees: Who's the Boss?

" You can employ men and hire hands to work for you, but you must win their hearts to have them work with you "

William H.H. Boetcker

Even though many entrepreneurs start their businesses single-handedly, it would be very difficult (and probably not a good idea) for a nurse practitioner to do so. You need at least one employee, if not two. You need to have a live person answering the telephone during regular business hours. Chances are that if you rely on voice mail or other recording devices you will lose more patients than you gain. Selecting the best employee can be the most important business decision you make. When dealing with potential employees and existing employees, try to be mindful of employment laws. You should schedule some time with your legal advisor to go over the "do's and don'ts" in hiring before you start the process if you are not knowledgeable on the current laws.

STAFFING

Depending on the type of practice you design, the number of employees you need to hire will vary. You may work well with just one employee or you may need to add others. Just remember, with every employee comes the expenses (salary, taxes, insurance) of the employee. You don't want to overextend yourself in the early months of business. Part-time or per-diem employees may be helpful during your busier hours. Be flexible with your staffing. With every position you create, you must write out the responsibilities for that position. These can be changed, but initially you need them to give the potential employee a clear picture of what is expected.

You may have some experience already with managing employees; however, managing employees in your own business is a lot different. There is a delicate balance to maintain—you want to have a happy staff, but still have control and be productive. You want to make your employees feel important and that their input is valuable. Remember your favorite supervisor or manager from your past? What are the qualities of that manager that you admired? How would you handle people differently? You want to create a family atmosphere while maintaining the "head of the household" role. You do not want to be perceived as a dictator, but as more of a team leader.

To create this "team feeling," devise some productivity incentives such as offering a bonus. Whether it is a percentage of your revenues at the end of the year or a certain dollar amount if you reach a certain goal, you will certainly have your employee's attention by offering a bonus. Reinforce the message that the employee profits when the practice profits. This helps tie them into cost-cutting practices and collections. To maximize your potential revenues, it is key to carefully match your employees to the different tasks, design workflow systems, communicate your goals, and celebrate success. Efficient service from your employees is the goal. This will help build your practice by keeping the patients satisfied, while freeing you up to see more patients.

Respectful relationships between you and your staff as well as among the staff members is key for employee retention and increased production. Work on creating and maintaining a positive work environment—it will benefit you, your patients, employees, and your business. Keep morale high! Make your employees feel special and appreciated. If you feel the mood of the office isn't good, address it with your staff, get to the root of the problem. Then, take them all to lunch!

EMPLOYEE VERSUS INDEPENDENT CONTRACTOR

Some employers are eager to call their employees "independent contractors," and when you look at the financial benefits of using an independent contractor you will understand why. Businesses save large sums of money by not having to pay the independent contractor the required federal taxes, state taxes, unemployment taxes, and Social Security that must be paid to employees.

Owners gain great benefits by distinguishing between employees and independent contractors; however, the business owner must be aware that the Internal Revenue Service (IRS) looks closely at independent contractor classifications. If the IRS finds that the independent contractor does not fit the criteria, then they can reclassify the employee retroactively and collect payment, essentially wiping out the profits of the business and causing it to fold, or bringing criminal penalties against the owner. The IRS has produced a classification test to help determine whether your prospective employee should be an employee or an independent contractor. See Figure 13–1 for the 20-point classification test for independent contractors.

FINDING THE PERFECT EMPLOYEE

Selecting the right candidate for your employment position is always a challenge. To make the best selection, first define the expected duties of the employee by creating a job description. List the special knowledge, skills, qualifications, and physical requirements of the position. Then, simply write the basic tasks of the position (e.g., answering telephones, scheduling appointments, weighing the patients). Be as thorough as possible. Have the candidate read the written job description before the beginning of the interview. This step will ensure that all applicants receive the same information on the requirements for the position. If this position is going to require special skills such as performing phlebotomy, that will help narrow your search. Employers sometimes think that if they hire smart people, the employees will be able to figure out what to do. The pitfall is that smart people might come up with directions for themselves that are not in line with your business strategy. All employees need some guidance. Clearly communicate job expectations to the job applicant. The job description doesn't have to be set in stone; just make sure that conversations about expectations continue as the position evolves.

Now that you know what you require, you can start advertising for the position. Besides the local newspaper, local schools, and bulletin boards, check with others in the same position at other offices. Many times, employees from other offices may know of potential employees who are in-between jobs. If you are willing to train an employee, the local trade schools may give you leads on new graduates to interview. However, an experienced employee may prove beneficial during your first years of your practice.

Before you start the interviewing process, do a little research. Find out how much is the going rate for this type of position. You will want to decide what you can afford and what is a realistic salary. Have a salary range in mind, work it out in both hourly and annual amounts so you will have the correct figures in front of you when discussing salary during the interview.

While you are doing your research, you may want to check out what the other offices are providing as far as benefits are concerned. Know the costs and know what you can and cannot provide.

STEPS TO A SUCCESSFUL INTERVIEW

The interviewer should review the candidate's application and resume before the scheduled interview. Evaluate the application for neatness, completeness,

Figure 13-1	**Independent Contractor's Classification Test**

	Yes	No
• Is the individual experienced, qualified and available to do the work for the general public?	☐	☐
• Does the individual determine the manner in which the work is accomplished?	☐	☐
• Will the individual have to receive any training from the company?	☐	☐
• Is the individual responsible for all taxes, including federal, state, local, Social Security, and disability?	☐	☐
• Will the individual use his or her own facilities, equipment, and supplies?	☐	☐
• Will the individual be paid in a lump sum?	☐	☐

A "yes" answer to the above questions suggests that the individual is probably correctly classified as an independent contractor.

	Yes	No
• Will you pay the individual hourly wages, percentages of the profits, commission, or salary?	☐	☐
• Do you exercise any supervision over the individual's work other than acceptance or rejection of the final product?	☐	☐
• Do you have any responsibility to employ or pay helpers or assistants for the individual?	☐	☐
• Do you guarantee the individual a minimum amount of compensation for the work?	☐	☐
• Is the individual required to keep an expense account or travel log?	☐	☐
• Do you provide the individual with a permit or license or pay for the same if it required for the individual to do the work?	☐	☐

A "yes" answer to the above questions suggests that the individual is probably not correctly classified as an independent contractor.

and accuracy. Make notes if information is missing or if there are gaps in the employment history and education sections. Look for a history of job stability and professional growth.

You should prepare interview questions before you start the interview process. You can start with jotting down the questions that were raised when you read the application and the resume. During the interview, you can give hypothetical situations and ask how the candidate would handle the situation—you can write those out before hand as well. Pay attention to the answers given for inconsistencies, and pay attention to the applicant's eye contact, speech, and body language.

You also should ask about their skills and abilities. Where did they get any additional training? Ask about their career goals and objectives—short- and long-term goals. Questions about their academic programs and achievements as well as their work experiences should give you good information. Ask about their accomplishments and achievements.

The appearance of the applicant can give you more information about the potential employee's habits and attention to detail. Is the person neat and clean with clean nails and appropriate hair? Are his or her clothes clean and in good repair? Are there any visible piercings or tattoos? Did the candidate arrive on time for the interview? Would you feel comfortable with this person representing you in your office and the community? Good social skills are very important when dealing with patients and other professionals. Depending on your situation, you may choose an employee with better social skills over the employee with better technical skills. Maturity, personality, common sense, and the ability to follow directions are important characteristics to identify during the interview process.

Interview notes should be written on a separate piece of paper, not on the application form. Sign and date the end of the interview notes. Avoid writing things about personal characteristics (race, age, personality). After the position has been filled, you should put in writing on each interview note why the individual was not selected. Be sure to use legitimate, nondiscriminatory reasons for the rejection.

You must have a system for interviews and background checks for hiring your staff, because any misbehavior of your staff not only reflects on your practice but also can lead to future lawsuits. Call a couple of the job references given on the application. You may learn some things that could prevent major problems for your practice. You may even want to go to the expense of having a professional background check performed. You do want to know whether the applicant has a history of stealing, don't you? In this age of the Internet you can learn a lot about your prospective employee. There are several Internet businesses that will perform the check for a nominal fee (e.g., *www.repchceck.com, www.knowx.com, www.informus.com,* and *www.confi-chek.com*). Laws regarding what information an employer can and cannot consider vary among the states. You may also need to get written consent from the potential employee to perform the background check. State laws also address what a past employer can and cannot say about a former employee. Know the law.

Are you considering hiring one of your children to do some filing or cleaning? Information regarding child labor laws is available at *www.dol.gov*. There are tax benefits to doing this. The wages you pay your child count as a deductible business expense for you. That reduces your taxable income. If the child is younger than 18 and your business is a sole proprietorship, your child's wages are exempt form Social Security and Medicare taxes. Be sure to check this out with your accountant before you hire your child.

EFFECTIVELY NEGOTIATING SALARY AND BENEFITS

The negotiation phase of the interview can be fun and interesting. The specifics to discuss at this time include salary, hours, bonus compensation, non-compete clauses, benefits, and future compensation increases.

Usually there is a place on the application form for the applicant to state an expected salary. This should give you a starting point for discussion. If the applicant uses the words "open," "negotiable," or "competitive," ask him or her "What are your salary requirements?" If the answer is vague, then ask how much the person earned at his or her last job. Have a range in mind, but be flexible. You can always delay making a decision for a few days. Ask the applicant what benefits are most important. You can also check the applicant's past salary history on the application. Be sure to take good notes.

You have specific needs, demands, wishes, and requirements for your prospective employee. Think them through and discuss them openly with the applicant. Remember, this discussion about salary is usually a stressful part of the interview for the applicant. You can use this time to gather information from the applicant. If the applicant requires more than what you are prepared to offer, you may consider adding to the job responsibilities, such as cleaning the office, going to the post office, or going to the grocery to buy supplies for the office kitchen. These extra duties may help justify a higher wage.

In addition to the salary, the applicant will be weighing out the benefits package as well. Some of the basics most employers provide include:

- Health insurance
- Paid vacation
- Paid sick leave
- Paid holidays

A more comprehensive package might include:

- Life insurance
- Dental insurance
- Optical insurance
- Bonuses

- Child care and daycare services
- Company car
- Tuition reimbursement
- Cost-of-living adjustments
- Disability insurance
- Malpractice insurance
- Continuing education costs
- Expense accounts
- Flexible work schedule
- Maternity/parental leave
- Parking
- Professional membership dues
- Profit sharing programs
- Retirement plans
- Savings plans
- Special equipment
- Unpaid personal leave time

EMPLOYMENT AGREEMENT

An employment agreement is a legal contract that spells out the conditions of a working relationship between an employer and an employee. You may choose not to use employment agreements or contracts with your employees. It is your decision. It seems that no matter how the contract is written, if the employee doesn't want to work with you—he or she won't. If you do opt to use an employment contract, make sure it is up to date and accurately identifies the areas of responsibility. Trouble can arise when employees do not clearly understand their responsibilities and duties.

Employment contracts usually contain the following basic components:

- A listing of the general duties expected from the employee
- A listing of the employee's salary and benefits
- The duration of the contract (usually 1 year)
- Contract review time frame (usually annually)
- Amendment and modification agreement (only with both parties' signatures)
- Termination of contract conditions
- Restrictive clause if they do not complete the contract
- Signatures with date and names printed

This contract should be prepared with the guidance of your legal advisor. With the advice and counsel of your legal advisor, develop an employee handbook. This will help you and the employee. Have clear definitions as well as firm policies outlined. Determine and implement procedures to comply with the state and federal requirements.

EMPLOYER RESPONSIBILITIES

Now that you have completed your search and found your new employee, you need to uphold your promises and obligations. As an employer, you have some legal responsibilities. First, you need to verify American citizenship or legal immigration status. You need to have a copy of the documents on file. A copy of the employee's Social Security card and driver's license should be kept in a personnel file as well. You must comply with the provisions of the Americans with Disabilities Act. That information can be found at *www.usdoj.gov/crt/ ada/adahom1.htm*.

If your employee has a professional license or certification, you should keep a copy of it on file. If it has an expiration date, note that on your calendar so you can keep current copies. You are responsible for ensuring the safety of your patients by making sure your employees are adequately trained. You are also responsible for providing a safe working environment for your employees. You must withhold and pay the appropriate taxes. If worker's compensation insurance is required, you must pay for it. Unemployment insurance premiums must be paid for your employees. Make arrangements to fulfill all of your promises for benefits.

Take the time to properly orient and train your new employees. It is better to let them know what you expect from the beginning rather than having to correct their mistakes. Even the simplest task of answering the telephone should be addressed. Let your new employees know exactly how you would like them to answer the telephone.

Let your new employees know when you plan on reviewing their performance—will it be in 3 months, 6 months, or even a year? Put the date on the calendar, then follow through with the meeting. Employees want to know where they stand. They need to hear about the things they are doing well as well as the areas where they need improvement.

PREVENTING WORKPLACE VIOLENCE

There is an average of 970,000 reported violent incidences annually in workplaces in the United States (U.S. Department of Justice report, 1995). As the employer, you may be responsible for the safety of every person in your office—employees, patients, and members of the public. Workplace violence should be addressed in the employee handbook—zero tolerance should be enforced for both violence and sexual harassment.

Workplace violence affects your business's profitability—including medical or disability benefits, psychological counseling for victims and survivors, and repair of property damage. Other costs involved with workplace violence include lost productivity and potential liability.

The first step in prevention of workplace violence is to be cautious when hiring employees. Company policies must clearly state that inappropriate behavior in the workplace, such as violence or threatening behavior, is a ground for immediate termination. But policies and handbooks are not enough; employers need to take all threats seriously and investigate them immediately.

The fact that you have a medical office may lead to attempted break-ins or robberies during or after your office hours. Thieves may be looking for drugs, money, or your office equipment. Depending on your setting, you may want to have an alarm company install a panic button at the front desk. Develop a plan for your receptionist to carry out if a suspicious person enters the office, including having a special code that puts everyone on alert. Some clinics that have been threatened or have experienced violence have gone so far as to install not only a panic button but also bullet-proof glass separating the employees from the waiting room. Hopefully, you will not ever have to deal with violence in your workplace, but it is better to be prepared.

Prevention is the key to dealing with potential workplace violence. Discuss with your employees how you would like them to handle certain violent scenarios. Brainstorm on how to make the office safer for all of you. Remind your employees to be on alert for potential violence and suspicious behavior and to report it to you before it exacerbates into a tragedy. Know your patients and alert your staff if you feel there is potential for danger.

If a threat of violence or actual violence occurs in your office, you must report it to the police immediately. Get medical attention and counseling for your employees as necessary. After the situation has been resolved, sit down in a quiet room and write down your account of the event with as many details as possible. Include the names of all parties involved (victims, perpetrators, and witnesses). Also, include any environmental factors. If there is a crime scene you may want to photograph it for your records. Be sure to put the time and date on the document and then sign it. Put this document in a safe place. As you know, with time, personal accounts of some events change. This could prove to be a valuable document. Maintaining a safe environment for your employees is *your* responsibility.

SUGGESTIONS AND TIPS FROM WOMEN'S HEALTH WATCH, INC.

When negotiating with my first employee, she stated that she needed $2 more per hour than I had budgeted. We found a way to make it work. Instead of hiring a cleaning company to come in to the office, she would do the work. Once a week, she did a thorough cleaning (and I mean thorough!) and kept the place immaculate throughout the week. For this wonderful service, I cheerfully paid the extra $2 per hour.

PERSONAL ANECDOTES

1. I am very fortunate in that my office manager has wonderful social skills as well as great experience working in a medical office. She has taught me a lot. We do make jokes about "Who is really the boss here?" It seems that we take turns! It works well for us since I trust her implicitly.

2. We have such a wonderful friendship as well as a great working relationship. On the days when the schedule permits, we start the day with a cup of coffee and we do the crossword puzzle together (actually, we both race through it trying to finish before the other!). What a great way to start the day!

Resources

American Hospital Association: Creating a secure workplace: Effective policies and practices in healthcare: *www.aha.org/resource/onlinecatalog.asp.*

Americans with Disabilities Act: *www.usdoj.gov/crt/ada/adahom1.htm.*

Background check companies: *www.repchceck.com, www.knowx.com, www.informus.com, and www.confi-chek.com.*

Buppert, C: Employment agreements: Clauses that can change an NP's life. Nurse Pract 22(8):108–119, 1997.

Child labor laws: *www.dol.gov.*

Duke, D: A legal look at hiring—Part 1. Nurs Spectrum 12, 5:6–7, 2000.

Gilmore-Hall, A: Violence in the workplace. Am J Nursing 101:7, 2001.

Kristof, K: Straight answers. Family Money 14:7, 2000.

Larkin, H: Get the most from staff and ancillaries. Medical Economics Magazine [online, 1999] 11,1: *http://www.pdr.net/memag/static.htm?path=docs/011199/article4.html.*

OSHA Guidelines for preventing workplace violence for health care and social service workers: 202-693-1888 or *www.osha.gov.*

Rosenberg, JA, and Owens, P: Top 10 resolutions for CEO's. Enterprising Women 10, 2:34–35, 2001.

Sample employment contract: The 2001 Sourcebook for Advanced Practice Nurses 5,1, 2001.

Starr, DS: Tips for everyday clinical practice: The freestanding practitioner. Clin Advisor 24, 4:121, 2000.

Workplace violence, can you close the door on it? (Brochure) American Nurses Association: 1-800-274-4ANA *or www.nursingworld.org.*

N O T E S

Chapter 14

Patient Communication: I Have to Keep Them Happy!

" People will forget what you said. People will forget what you did...But people will never forget how you made them feel "

Anonymous

Your communication skills can make or break your practice. Good people skills are a must. These are skills that can be learned and practiced. As your confidence as a provider grows, you may notice your communication with your patients will become easier as well. Not only are good communication skills good for patient relations, but your business will also benefit.

CUSTOMER CARE

It has been said, "It takes months to find a customer...Seconds to lose one." All the marketing in the world will not help your practice if you and your staff are not customer oriented. Patients need to feel they are important—not just another patient squeezed into the nurse practitioner's busy schedule. You want to create a collegial feeling between you and the patient—working together to better the patient's health.

From the first telephone call to your office, throughout the appointment, to the time they walk out the door—you want your patients to feel welcome, comfortable, and satisfied. With the right person answering the telephone and greeting the patient, you can start things off on the right foot. You want a friendly office atmosphere, creating an egalitarian feeling for the patient. The patient should be made to feel comfortable in asking questions. Patients also want information on what they can be doing themselves to enhance their health.

McCall's magazine featured a list of "8 Reasons to Switch Doctors." That list included the following:

1. He always seems to keep me waiting.
2. I call and call… and never hear back.
3. I never get to finish what I'm saying.
4. She blows off my questions.
5. He acts as if I don't know anything.
6. He refuses to make enough time for me.
7. We just don't see things eye to eye.
8. I can't trust her to get things right.[1]

You should treat your patients in the manner that you want and expect your family to be treated when they visit their health care provider. No matter how busy you are, sit down, look your patients in the eye, let them talk, and give them your undivided attention. If your patients feel like they're not improving, make it evident that you are on their side and you will help them through their problems.

Carry out your promises. If you say you will call a patient, be sure to make the call, even if you don't have what you thought you would (such as test results or referrals). Give your patients an update and don't let them feel forgotten. Taking the time to call and check on a patient is time well spent. Patients truly appreciate and value the attention. Pay attention to what your customers want. Your customers are your patients, their families, and their referring physicians. Never be too rushed to be polite. Take good care of all of your customers and you will certainly do well.

Investigate whether or not your state has published a "Patient's Bill of Rights and Responsibilities." If there is one published for your state, you should read it and possibly post it in your office. Hopefully, this publication will seem redundant, in that you already recognize and respect your patient's rights. For an example, refer to the *Summary of the Florida Patient's Bill of Rights and Responsibilities*, which can be accessed through the Website *http://www.doh.state.fl.us/mqa/profiling/billofrights.htm*. Some practitioners in Florida have their patients initial a copy of this document before any procedures are performed, which may be helpful if a lawsuit develops. A national patient's bill of rights may eventually be instituted. Because providing health care is viewed less as an art and more as a business, those who run the business must pay more attention to the needs of their customers.

Be sure to give 100 percent of your attention to your patient once you shut the exam room door. Instruct your staff not to interrupt you unless for an emergency. Patients expect and deserve your undivided attention. A purely medical approach that ignores prevention, healthy lifestyles, and patient selfcare is not comprehensive health care. Keep your nursing foundation in your practice.

TELEPHONE COMMUNICATION

Good quality telephone equipment is imperative to good telephone communication. You cannot have a successful conversation over a crackling line that disconnects itself. So, you will want to have the best system you can easily afford installed. Be sure you maintain a sufficient number of telephone lines to enable patients to get through to the office without getting a busy signal. Choose a system that allows expansion as your business grows. Using an intercom system within the telephone system produces a much more professional impression than having someone yell down the hall "You have a call on line one!"

Decide how to handle after-hours telephone calls. There are many sophisticated systems that can transfer the call to your cell phone or even beep you. It may be more appropriate for you to hire an answering service. If you are not available for after-hours care, you must be careful how you word your message on your answering machine. You may want to call around to local medical offices to hear how the competition's calls are being handled. If you use voice mail, listen to your own message. Make sure it is upbeat and concise. If you have any type of automated telephone system, make sure there is a way to reach a real person immediately during office hours.

Think about how you want your prospective patients to be greeted on the telephone. Write it out for your staff. Take the time to train them to speak the way you want to be represented. It is good to have them include their name in the greeting. It makes the call more personal, and your staff members will be more accountable if the patient knows their name. If your staff does not sound friendly when answering the telephone, you must address the issue. One technique some professionals use is to have a small mirror on their desk and to speak while smiling at themselves. It creates a much nicer sounding voice. Your staff needs to exude a caring attitude through the telephone. How nice it is to hear "I came to you because the lady on the telephone was so nice to me!" Hopefully, you will hear that comment over and over.

Make sure that when telephone calls are transferred to other extensions, an explanation is given to the caller of what is being done. Try to avoid putting callers immediately on hold when they call the office. If a patient call must be put on hold, then have your staff make sure the patient is taken care of quickly. Be sure to return telephone calls in a timely manner.

Devise a foolproof system for receiving telephone messages from your staff. A simple notepad next to the telephone can be used for writing messages, and you can return those calls when you're available. Traditional telephone message pads can be used, the messages can be clipped to the patient's chart, and the chart can be held in a specific location. However you decide to handle your messages, make sure that you receive all the telephone messages and that you return your calls as soon as possible. More than one lawsuit has cited a provider for not calling back the patient in a timely fashion. Don't let this happen to you.

Give your staff a thorough training on how to triage telephone calls. Write out specific instructions and keep updating the instructions. Let them know what the major signs of danger to your patients include (e.g., difficulty breathing, chest pain, rapid heart beats). Develop procedures with your staff regarding calls from hospitals, health care providers, nursing homes, pharmacies, and the like. Don't just let your staff make these decisions. It is your practice, your reputation, your responsibility, and your license that is on the line.

APPOINTMENT SCHEDULING

As computers become more sophisticated and easy to use, more and more medical software is being developed. Some programs include appointment scheduling systems. This may help you with your time management; or it could be too cumbersome for your staff. If you use your computer for scheduling, you need always to have your computer turned on. If you are working in another computer program, you will have to save your information and exit that program before you can make a simple appointment.

Your office supply store carries appointment books. Check out their layout and choose one that you feel will work for you. Always have pencils near the appointment book. You will want to be able to adjust and change appointments written in the book.

Write out guidelines for your staff. Tell them specifically how many minutes to book for each type of exam and procedure you perform. You could write the number of minutes needed for each item on a copy of a superbill as a quick reference sheet. Also, write the cost of the visit or procedure on the same superbill so your staff can give correct information to patients. You might also want to write out what you want them to tell the patient after they have scheduled the appointment, for example, "We will see you on June 15th at 3 o'clock. Payment is due at the time of your appointment. We accept cash, MasterCard, and Visa. You will be seeing Carolyn Zaumeyer, nurse practitioner. Do you have any questions?"

As your practice grows, you will be able to refine your scheduling to make it work best for you and your patients. Many polls have shown that patients resent having to wait more than 15 minutes for an appointment and only 20% thought a 30-minute wait was acceptable.[2]

Have your staff keep patients in the waiting area updated on the schedule. If the nurse practitioner is running late, have the staff try to contact the patient before he or she leaves work or home to come to the office. Give the patient the option of rescheduling if the appointment is delayed. Give the patient the courtesy you would like extended to you.

Really think about how your staff should respond to insurance questions over the telephone. You really don't want your staff saying, "We don't take that insurance" and hanging up. An alternative is "We are not currently contracted with your insurance company; however, we'll be happy to work with your out-of-network coverage to make the finances easy for you." That way, you are not simply telling the patient to go elsewhere, rather you are offering an option for the patient to see you.

PATIENT EDUCATION

Patient education is a fundamental part of nursing care. Patient education should be the core component of every nurse practitioner's role—not just for the patient, but also for the families when appropriate. A good goal may be for your patient to leave your office with three new bits of health knowledge. If you can give the patients literature to take home, they may be able to really learn the new information.

There are many sources for preprinted patient education sheets. Many journals now incorporate patient education sheets into articles that you can copy and hand out to your patients. The pharmaceutical representatives are a good resource for patient materials. Your specialty organizations may also have patient handouts. You can have customized patient information or custom practice brochures designed and printed. One company that provides this service is Contemporary Health Communications at 1-800-234-1742 or *http://patient-info.com*. If you cannot find a patient education sheet for a certain disorder, procedure, or medication, you can easily create one on your computer and then have copies made for distribution.

Patients do appreciate the extra effort you take in providing them information. Many patients want to know more about health promotion, and this is a great way to pass on good information. You can also pass on some Website addresses to your patients that you feel might give them more information. Some Websites that might be appropriate for your patients include:

- Medline*plus* at *http://www.medlineplus.gov.*
- National Institutes of Health at *www.nih.gov/health.*
- Office on Women's Health at *www.4women.gov.*
- Mayo Clinic at *www.mayoclinic.com.*
- National Library of Medicine at *www.nlm.nih.gov.*
- Columbia University "Go ask Alice" at *www.goaskalice.columbia.edu.*
- U.S. Department of Health at *www.healthfinder.gov.*
- National Center for Complementary and Alternative Medicine at *http://nccam.nih.gov.*
- National Headache Foundation at *www.headaches.org.*
- National Institute of Mental Health at *www.nimh.nih.gov.*
- The American Autoimmune Related Disease Association at *www.aarda.org.*

You can also take advantage of the waiting area in your office by displaying literature and even running videos on fitness and health. Be sure to document the educational materials you provide to your patient. It may be helpful if a lawsuit develops.

DRUG ADVERTISEMENTS

Over the past several years, direct advertisements to the public by the pharmaceutical companies has increased significantly. How do you handle the patient who comes in with an advertisement and demands a prescription for that specific medication? What if the medication is not the best treatment for the patient? What if the advertised medication is not included in their insurance formulary? Every situation is different. However, there are some basic guidelines in being able to keep your patient happy and being able to continue to give the best care possible.

First, show patients you care by letting them talk; let them tell you why they feel this medication is good for them. Don't get defensive. After you let them tell you why they feel this medication is appropriate, acknowledge their initiative for bringing in the drug information. After all, they are trying to become active and involved in their own health care. In a neutral tone (you don't want to start an argument), review the options available. Let each patient decide which option to choose. Be sure to document this conversation well. So, the basic steps are to (1) establish empathy, (2) gather information, and (3) hold your recommendations until the end.[3] Patients are more likely to adhere to a treatment plan you both agree on; let the patient help design the plan.

PATIENT PRIVACY AND CONFIDENTIALITY

Your entire staff must be acutely aware of the importance of maintaining the privacy and confidentiality of all patient information. You must teach your staff members the importance of privacy and confidentiality as soon as they are hired. You may want to set a strict policy that states that if any information is released inappropriately then the persons responsible will be terminated. This is a very serious issue. Gossip about patients should not be tolerated. Explain to your staff how friends or family members of patients may overhear conversations that could result in complaints of breach of patient confidentiality that eventually may lead to a lawsuit. Be sure that billing matters are also discussed in private.

Watch and listen to how your staff interacts with your patients. Do they ask out loud in front of others "What's your problem?" or something along those lines? Staff members should take patients into another room or out of hearing distance of other patients to discuss the reason for their appointment. Remember, you want patients to feel comfortable in your office.

Know the federal and state laws regarding patient privacy. Know what information you can release and to whom. Know which records require written consent for release from the patient. Know which records can be faxed and which records cannot be faxed. Know the patient's rights. If you do not follow the regulations, you may face monetary fines up to $250,000 and 10 years in jail![4]

In the year 2000, the Department of Health and Human Services (HHS) issued the final regulations on medical records privacy under the Health Insurance Portability and Accountability Act (HIPAA) of 1996. The privacy regulations involve many areas, including, among others, how patients receive notice of their rights, how providers obtain patient information needed for treatment, patient authorizations, and disclosure of patient information to insurance companies. To learn more about patient privacy, contact the United States Department of Health and Human Services at *www.hhs.gov/ocr/ hipaa.html* or other helpful Websites including *www.hipaadvisory.com* and *www.healthprivacy.org.*

TERMINATION OF THE PROVIDER/PATIENT RELATIONSHIP

There may come a time when the termination of the provider/patient relationship cannot be avoided. Be sure you have a credible reason for the dismissal. You do not want the dismissal to appear to be based on discrimination of any sort. There are specific guidelines for severing this relationship. If the proper steps are not followed, you may be charged with abandonment. Before the relationship is terminated, the medical status of the patient must be evaluated, documented, and, if applicable, the patient should be referred to your collaborating physician. If the patient belongs to a managed care plan, you must know what steps to follow to have the patient reassigned to another provider. If you do not follow the managed care plans rules, you may be in violation of your contract.

Remember that patients have well-defined rights. The Patient's Bill of Rights is very detailed and includes the patient's right to choose a provider. Be sure to know what is stated in the Patient's Bill of Rights (*http://thomas. loc.gov*).

To dismiss a patient, you must notify him or her in writing on your letterhead and you should mail the letter by certified mail with return receipt requested. Malpractice insurers provide sample letters, but they suggest that the letters be modified according to the circumstances. Some insurers want a specific reason for the dismissal, whereas others believe it is better not to give specifics. A sample dismissal letter can be viewed at *http://me.pdr.net/me/*

content/journals/m/data/2000/0410/screen/m4a05401.jpg. Offer to forward the medical records promptly to the new provider of choice once you receive written authorization. Send only copies; keep the originals in your office. Make sure the appointment scheduler knows about the termination of the patient and what to say if the patient calls to schedule an appointment with you. Give the patient at least 30 days' notice before the relationship is terminated. This timeframe can be extended if the patient is unable to find a new provider. If the patient refuses to accept the certified letter, file the returned unopened letter in the patient's chart and then send another letter by regular mail. Document in the chart when the second letter was sent. Hopefully, you may never be faced with this situation, but it is good to know how to handle it if the situation does arise.

SUGGESTIONS AND TIPS FROM WOMEN'S HEALTH WATCH, INC.

- For telephone messages, we kept a yellow legal pad at the front desk. All of the messages from the answering machine and when I was out of the office were recorded on this pad with the date and time. When I arrived at the office, I reviewed the messages with my office manager. If there were any urgent messages, I took care of them immediately. Once the calls were returned, I made a check mark next to the message indicating the call was returned. Having the messages all in one place made it easy for my staff when I called to ask whether there were any messages. This log also was helpful if we needed to locate a telephone number later that we knew was recorded on the pad. It was also helpful to have the messages recorded with the date and time.

- How you handle the release of patient medical records can be tricky. Some patients demand to have a copy for themselves, whereas others are happy if you forward them on to a provider or insurance company. Be sure not to release the records without the patient's signature on a records release form. We had an office policy that no records left the office without my approval. I put a distinctive mark on the pages that were to be released. That saved my staff the responsibility of deciding what needed to be sent and what didn't. We also knew by looking for the mark which papers had left the office.

PERSONAL ANECDOTE

I am so fortunate with my office staff. My office manager has such a good ear; she can recognize most of our regular patients by their voice over the telephone! They are amazed and flattered. She greets them by name when they walk in the door and she remembers special things about the patients. She is amazing. Hopefully, you will find a "right hand" person as wonderful as mine. It makes life at work a lot easier and a lot more fun having someone so clever around!

Resources

Brown, D: On-the-job etiquette. BJ's Journal (Fall) 25:22–23, 2000.

Carnegie, D: Managing through people. New York: Dale Carnegie and Associates, 1999.

Contemporary Health Communications: 1-800-234-1742 or *http://patient-info.com.*

Crane, M: How to cut loose from a troublesome patient. Medical Economics [online, April 10, 2000] 3: *http://www.pdr.net/memag/public.htm?path = docs/041000/ article3.html.*

Dismissal sample letter—*http://me.pdr.net/me/content/journals/m/data/2000/ 0410/screen/m4a05401.jpg.*

Grandinetti, D: What kind of patient would rather see a nurse practitioner? Medical Economics [online, February 8, 1999], 4: *http://www.pdr.net/memag/static.htm? path = docs/020899/article4.html.*

HIPAA Advisory: *www.hipaadvisory.com*

Leawood, KS: Patient education in your practice: A handbook for the office setting. American Academy of Family Physicians, 1999.

Mason, DJ: Promoting health literacy. American Journal of Nursing (February) 101:7, 2001.

Medline*plus*: *http://www.medlineplus.gov.*

Miller, SK: What are your rights regarding patient selection? Patient Care for the Nurse Practitioner 9(50), 2001.

Slomski, AJ: "Boutique" practices: Good medicine—or ethical swamp? Medical Economics [online, July 24, 2000] 5: *http://www.pdr.net/memag/ public.htm?path = docs/article5.html.*

Starr, DS: HIPAA's new privacy standards. Clin Advisor 101:5, 2001.

Summary of the Florida Patient's Bill of Rights and Responsibilities *http://www.doh.state.fl.us/mqa/profiling/billofrights.htm.*

United States Department of Health and Human Services: *www.hhs.gov/ocr/hipaa.html.*

References

1. Laliberte, R: 8 Reasons to switch doctors. McCall's (May) 79:78–80, 2000.
2. Cotterell, Mitchell & Fifer, Inc: Nurse practitioner risk management procedure guide. New York: PractitionerCare, 1997.
3. Lowes, R: "Doc, I saw this great new drug on TV..." Medical Economics [online, April 26, 1999] 3: *http://www.pdr.net/memag/static.htm?path = docs/042699/ article3.html.*
4. Knopper, M: Protecting patient privacy. Clinician News (March) 3:1–9, 2001.

N O T E S

Chapter 15

Increasing the Revenues: How Can We Make More Money?

" Everything can be improved "

C. W. Barron

Successful business owners are constantly looking for creative ways to increase their productivity, with the goal of increasing their business's revenues. Because we are all coming from an altruistic nursing background, this may be a difficult concept for some of us to accept. To put this in perspective, you must lay your nursing cap aside for a few moments and put on your business hat. If your practice is not producing enough income to cover the expenses of the practice, you will not have a practice very long. You need to find a way not only to cover the expenses of your practice, but also to provide yourself with a comfortable income.

You must take as good of care of your business as you do of your patients. This is all possible without compromising your ethical standards. Just as you do not practice outside your scope of practice, do not do or sell anything that you do not truly believe in. The last thing you want to do is compromise your reputation with your patients and the community. However, there are many good ways to help increase your practice's profitability.

EVALUATE YOUR CURRENT PRACTICE

Before you start adding different services and products to your practice, take a few moments and review what you are doing now. A few questions you may want to ask yourself include:

249

- Are you being paid appropriately for your time and efforts?
- Are your charges current?
- How about collections?
- Are you marking your charge slips for all appropriate charges?
- Do you have the right employee handling coding and collections?
- Are you coding with the most specific codes?
- Are you marketing your practice appropriately?
- Are you or your staff being wasteful with office and medical supplies?
- Are you getting a full day's work from your staff?
- Is there any way someone could be embezzling from your practice's finances?
- Are you giving away services or products needlessly?
- Is there any way to reduce the overhead or improve the productivity of your practice?

By answering the above questions, you may find some areas of your practice that could be easily improved upon that would lead to a more profitable practice. By reviewing your charges and your system of indicating to the billing staff what should be charged, you may find you are not collecting what is due to you. Inept coding could be doing your practice in. Not paying attention to your practice's accounts receivable (what is owed to you) can bleed your practice of its economic vitality.

To help you with this evaluation, pull 10 charts randomly; review the notes and the charges. Do they mesh? Were all of the services provided charged for appropriately? Is there room for improvement? You may want to do this exercise on a monthly basis, so you know exactly what is going on with your billing practices.

You should know exactly what your collectables are on a weekly basis. Do not simply leave this area of work to your staff. Keep tabs on what is owed and step in when needed to help with the collections.

ADVERTISING SPECIALS

People love a bargain. Don't you? Compile a promotion or package that you can advertise that will bring in people that may eventually become long-time patients. A testing package appropriate for your practice may help bring in patients, for example: "HIV, syphilis, chlamydia, and gonorrhea testing, all for only $75!" or "Free Pap smears Saturday from 9 until noon". Find a niche, something special that does not cost you a lot to bring in patients who otherwise may not have noticed your practice. In many communities, coupons are very well received. A simple $5 or $10 off the patient's charges may bring in many new patients. Don't be afraid to try something new or different.

WORKING IN ANOTHER PRACTICE SETTING

When first starting your practice, you may have some free time in your schedule. It may be beneficial to avail yourself to a part-time or per-diem work situation with another organization. Your income from other sources could help defray some of your practice's expenses. You might be able to use this time to market your own practice for referrals for services not performed within their practice (with the employer's permission, of course). Depending on the setting, you may have the opportunity to continue your growth clinically while working at another setting.

There are many employment opportunities for part-time or per-diem work situations. Many times, these opportunities are listed in the classified advertisements in the local newspaper. Potential employers include university student health centers, Planned Parenthood, physician's offices, public health centers, and urgent care or walk-in clinics.

PUBLIC SPEAKING

One of the best gifts you can give yourself and your practice is to become skilled at public speaking. Even if you are very shy, don't let that stand in your way. Being able to effectively speak and present information to a large group of people is very empowering. It can be terrifying as well as gratifying, but it is well worth the effort.

Public speaking can bring extra attention to you and your practice. Every time you speak at an event, you should send out a press release. If you include a picture of yourself, a professional "head shot" or a picture of you speaking at the event, chances are that your photo will be printed as well as your story! This of course brings added free publicity for you and your practice.

To get started, you need to assess your current public speaking skills. Do you know how to properly prepare and present a program? Have you developed a system for your notes so you can speak easily without reading? Can you design your own slide presentation? Have you ever been videotaped while speaking so you can evaluate your speech, appearance, and body language?

There are many different ways to train to become an effective public speaker. Some professional organizations help their members by providing speakers training courses at their meetings and conferences. One well-known and respected speakers training organization is *Toastmasters International*, which has chapters all over the world. For local chapter information, refer to their Website at *www.toastmasters.org*. Another training group you may want to investigate is *Speak Easy Seminars* (*www.speakeasy.net*). *Dale Carnegie* courses have been around for years and have helped a lot of people develop great communication and speaking skills (*www.westegg.com*).

Preparation is key to public speaking. If you are well prepared, you can have the confidence to stand in front of a group of people and be the "expert" on the subject you are presenting. With diligent research and planning, you can be confident that you know more about the topic you are presenting than any other person in the room.

Just as an essay has basic structure, good speeches follow specific structure as well. You should have a strong opening, a purposeful body, and a memorable conclusion. Once you have created the contents of your speech, you need to develop a system to keep you on track. Many speakers use cue cards to help them remember crucial data. Some speakers use a binder with an outline and reminders organized inside the binder. With time and practice, you will develop a system that will work for you.

The next step is practice, practice, and practice! Read over your speech out loud as many times as you can during the day, and then again right before you go to sleep at night. Fine-tune the wording so it flows easily. If there are specific words or sentences that give you difficulty, change them now! Get used to using your cue cards, slides, or your notes, as you will during your presentation. If you are not familiar or comfortable with the material you are presenting, you will be in trouble. Think of this as an area where you have control. You can research, plan, study, and learn your topic *before* you stand before your peers or the public as the expert. If you know your material, your self-confidence should be sky high! Concentrate on the material you are presenting instead of your own fears, and your nervousness will disappear. Relax and have fun!

The addition of slides to your presentation can really enhance your time in front of your audience. Microsoft's PowerPoint software is excellent for slide design and presentation. There are many "do's and don'ts" in slide design. You want the audience to be able to follow along and keep their interest in your presentation. The slides should be kept simple with the text large. For more tips on slide development, there are several books and CD-ROMs that can help you. One CD-ROM that is highly recommended is *Slides that Win* by Claudyne Wilder. She also offers a free e-newsletter *Presentation Points* available at *www.wilderpresentations.com*.

When you feel ready to speak publicly, search out opportunities. Your local and state nursing association meetings are a great place to start. You may see an advertisement in trade journals and newsletters entitled "Call for Abstracts." Organizations post these advertisements when they are planning educational meetings and need speakers. The organizations usually provide a very specific application for you to complete. If you have any questions or problems with the application, contact the sponsoring organization for help. You may also want to contact local clubs and organizations to offer your services to speak on your areas of expertise. The more experience you gain speaking, the more comfortable you will become speaking.

Once you have honed your speaking skills, you may want to avail yourself to the pharmaceutical companies related to your areas of practice and expertise. Many of the pharmaceutical companies have developed "speaker panels," and you may qualify to become a paid speaker for these companies. More speech tips can be found at *www.speechtips.com*, *www.toastmasters.rog/tips.htm*, and *www.angelfire.com/ab/speakers/checklist.htm*. This can be a fun and interesting way to increase revenues for your practice.

WRITING

It is doubtful that you have been able to attain a graduate degree without developing decent writing skills. Do you have an interest in writing? Does writing seem to come easy to you? Would you like to explore different opportunities in writing that may eventually lead to an increase in revenues for your practice? If so, do not hesitate to try your hand at writing professionally.

What subjects would you like to write about? Have you developed expertise in specific areas? Have you completed research that produced significant and interesting findings? Are you interested in sharing helpful information with your peers and the community? Honing your writing skills and having articles or books published can be very rewarding, not only financially and professionally, but also on a personal level.

Writing for your local nursing organization's newsletter is a great way to get started, and you will be helping out the organization as well. Your local newspaper may be looking for articles on health-related issues. Your articles may soon turn into a regular column. Once you get some experience and your confidence is high, your next step is to go on to the national magazines and journals.

Basic nursing magazines and nurse practitioner magazines are always looking for good writers. Continuing education articles are usually welcomed and the writers are usually rewarded with a nice compensation. Women's magazines and health magazines may be interested in articles written for the lay public. To locate contact information for your target media, simply look in the first few pages of the publication. Many have instructions printed inside for future writers. Be sure to do your homework before suggesting an article. Check the publication's prior issues for the past few years to make sure they have not recently published an article similar to the one you would like to propose. By reviewing prior articles, you can get an idea of the type of articles and the depth, style, and length of articles they publish. During the review, you may also identify subjects for more articles you could write.

Preparing a manuscript on a research project for publication has another set of challenges. There are specific rules to follow for each publication. Each journal differs in the type of manuscripts it accepts for publication. If you have an interest in this type of writing, look for the writer's guidelines in the journals you wish to target and follow the instructions to the letter.

Several nursing organizations offer mentoring programs for nurses interested in writing. The American Nurses Publishing (*www.nursesbooks.org*) has produced a free brochure *Guidelines for Authors* that maps out the process of publishing a book with them. They have also published a book *Writer's Guide to Nursing and Allied Health Journals* that is an excellent resource. This book contains valuable information on more than 600 journals, including all of the contact information for each journal.

The *Directory of Small Press/Magazine Editors and Publishers* lists the contact information for more of the mainstream monthly magazines. Publishing companies, such as F. A. Davis and American Nurse Publishing, often have opportunities available for nursing experts to review manuscript proposals. Many medical and nursing education organizations that provide continuing education for professionals have opportunities for new writers. One such organization, VISTAMedEd (VME), is an online medical and nursing education organization that provides continuing education to health care providers. They will provide you with a free *Vista Writer's Guide* (*www.vistameded.com*). They pay a competitive rate for manuscripts that are selected. Many times, there are advertisements in nursing magazines and journals for medical writers. NCLEX (*www.ncsbn.org*) also advertises for *item writers* to write questions for the NCLEX examination and for *item reviewers* to check the questions for currency, accuracy, job relatedness, and appropriateness for the entry-level nurse.

Writing a book can be a lot of fun and profitable as well. Good organizational skills are imperative for success. You first need to sketch out a rough outline and develop your concept. Fine-tune the outline, adding as much detail as possible. The outline can be changed as you go, but you should try to stick to the basic structure. Once you have firmed up your outline and concept, you may want to contact publishing companies that publish the type of book you are proposing. They can give you information on how to submit your proposal for publication. If publishing a book is a dream of yours, do yourself a big favor and follow through with your dream.

Writing articles and books can be very rewarding and can lead to endless wonderful opportunities. Writing can bring attention to you for your expertise and may lead to an increase in clientele and perhaps speaking engagements. You may be approached to write more on the subjects you have already written about or even to explore other areas. If you are having trouble planning an article or a book, just remember what the famous author Agatha Christie once said, "The best time for planning a book is while you're doing the dishes!"

TEACHING

In clinical practice you may have heard the saying "those who can do, do... Those who can't, teach!" Sounds like sour grapes from one who can do—but can't teach! If you get the opportunity to help guide a student to becoming a safe, confident, and competent health care provider, you should step up to the plate and give it your all. This can be a fantastic experience for both you and your students.

Many classes are scheduled in the evening, which means your clinical schedule may not be affected. Whether you will be teaching in the classroom, lab, or in the clinical area, you must get a detailed description of what is required of you. Then, you will be able to evaluate your responsibilities and project the time you will need to have available to complete your duties. Weigh out the salary against what they are asking of you. Is it worth it, or would your time be better spent in another area? Be sure to carefully look at the time required, to evaluate how this may affect your practice. If this experience is going to hurt your business in any way, don't do it. Remember, your business and the growth of your business are your first priority.

LEGAL CONSULTING

Some people have a true curiosity and attraction to legal matters. They watch all of the television shows about lawyers, court investigations, and the like. If you are one of those drawn to this area, you may want to consider becoming a legal consultant.

Legal consultants can work in court, providing expert testimony for lawsuits or investigating behind the scenes. There are many full and part-time positions available with law firms, insurance companies, government agencies, and health care providers for nurses with legal training.

Some of the duties of legal nurse consultants may include case summary, translation of medical records, standards of care definitions, verbal consultations with attorneys, testifying, and medical literature research.

There are several courses available for training to become a legal nurse consultant (LNC). Medical Legal Nurse Consulting Institute in Houston, Texas, offers a 6-week seminar for clinicians from around the country. Kaplan College offers a distance-learning program (*www.kaplancollege.edu/LN*). A correspondence course is available from Medical Litigation Review in Des Moines, Iowa, and another program is administered by the Florida Risk Management Institute via the Internet at *www.floridarisk.com* or 1-800-762-RISK.

Although certification is not required to work as a legal nurse consultant, national certification can be earned by examination through the American Association of Legal Nurse Consultants (*www.aalnc.org*).

DISPENSING PHARMACEUTICALS

It is estimated that more than 10 percent of physicians are now dispensing pharmaceuticals from their offices. The computerized dispensing systems have simplified the process of supplying and charging for prescription medications. The computers can communicate with insurance companies and HMOs for authorization for reimbursement, then actually dispense the medications while keeping an accurate inventory. There are monthly system and support charges, and a one-time licensing fee. Be sure to inquire of your licensing board regarding the legal aspects of nurse practitioners dispensing medications in your state before you make a commitment to the computer company. The potential increase in revenues with this system depends on the number of prescriptions you write. One company to contact for more information on this system is Tulsa-based Physicians Total Care at *www.physicanstotalcare.com* or 1-800-759-3650. It is probably best not to get involved in dispensing narcotics. Narcotics bring on their own set of problems of possible theft and abuse.

HOUSE CALLS

Nurse practitioners are leading the revival of house calls. One would think that geriatric patients would be the ideal patient base for home visits, but, depending on the situation, patients of all ages may benefit from house calls. The major advantage of a home visit is being able to assess the patient in his or her own environment. You can see firsthand the limitations that your patient faces every day.

The biggest challenge with house calls is getting reimbursed an amount that justifies the time spent on the visit, including your travel time. Your documentation must be very thorough, just as if you had seen the patient in your office. You also have the challenge of planning what equipment and supplies you will need to transport with you to the patient's home.

Making yourself available to all of the local hotels, motels, and other facilities for travelers could substantially increase your income. You may want to put together special marketing materials regarding house calls so the hotel management will have material to hand out and to refer to.

GRANTS

Many clinics and practices supplement their income with grants. The application process for grants can be tedious and overwhelming. Finding the right grant for your practice is a challenge, but something you may want to spend some time researching. The federal government (*www.fedmoney.com*) is a great place to start. One government site that specifically targets nurse practitioner practices can be found at *www.hrsa.gov/bhpr/grants.html*.

How nice it would be to receive a little extra money for providing your services to those covered in the grant. American Nurses Publishing (*www.nursesbooks.org*) has produced a great resource: *Grant Writing Tips for Nurses and Other Health Professionals* by Carol Kenner, DNS, RNC, FAAN, and

Marlene Walden, PhD, RNC, NNP. The faculty at your local nursing school may also be a good resource for assistance with grant writing. If you need more help completing the grant application, contact your local Small Business Association (SBA) office (*www.sba.gov*), which can guide you and possibly connect you with a mentor who can help you complete the grant application.

LEASING SPACE

Especially during your first year, there may be times when you are not using your office space. Why not lease it out and bring in some extra income? Some providers look to use an office in another location for a day or half a day per week to serve their patients in that area. There are different ways to determine the value of your space. Usually, interested providers have an idea of what they can pay. Sometimes, the payment is based on the time the space is used; other times, the payment is based on a percentage of the income collected during that time.

Before negotiating the use of your space, really think about the rules and limitations of your agreement. Will the provider be using your telephone, your copy machine, your lab supplies and equipment? Write it all down, so you both know exactly what you are agreeing to. A simple letter of agreement with the rules, limitations, and financial information documented should be sufficient to complete the deal. If you don't know the person or you are concerned about the deal, you could always have your attorney write up the agreement. How nice it is to have your location bringing in extra money when you aren't using it—Saturdays and evenings may be perfect for others to come in.

ACQUIRING NEW CLINICAL SKILLS

Whether you decide to start your own practice or continue to work in another setting, learning new clinical skills is essential for professional growth. Being able to provide comprehensive services for your patients is valuable both for the patient and your practice. Once you refer your patient outside of your practice for a procedure, you lose control of the quality of care given. When referring a patient for procedures, there may be a delay—either on the patient's part or on the part of the provider of the services. Learning new skills also makes you more marketable for future employers and insurance companies. Before you venture into new territory, make sure there are no legal restrictions preventing you from performing your new skill.

Assess your practice—try to identify skills or procedures that you don't currently include in your practice but you would like to add. Check with other practitioners within your specialty—see what they are doing that you are not. Professional educational meetings many times include skills training in which you can have an introduction to new skills. The calendars in nurse practitioner and medical journals may give you some ideas of available courses. The National Procedures Institute (NPI) offers many procedures and office surgery courses throughout the country. NPI can be contacted at *www.NPinstitute.com* or 1-800-462-2492. The books *Ambulatory Care Procedures for the Nurse Practitioner* by Margaret R. Colyar and Cynthia R. Ehrhardt and *Procedures for Nurse Practitioners* by Michael A. Carter have great information on office procedures. Some of the office procedures you may want to consider learning are listed in Figure 15–1.

Once you have completed a training course—whether it is a formal course or an informal one with another provider, design a system to record your performance. Document the dates of training and who provided the training. If possible, have the credentials of the trainer on file. Along with your instructor, you should create a log system with checks and balances to demonstrate your successful performance of the new skills. Take a moment and picture the worst case scenario: you in a court of law defending your self for performing this procedure. If your documentation system clearly shows your training, procedures completed, and successes, then you will have a strong defense. It is a better picture than one in which you say "I had some training a few years ago. I don't remember by whom, where, or when—then I just started doing the procedure on my own." I know that isn't a pleasant way to think, but it is better to be prepared than to practice in a cavalier manner. Learning new skills can be a fun and empowering way to increase your revenues.

SELLING PRODUCTS

It is no longer a rare occurrence to see products for sale in health care providers' offices. This practice has been met with mixed reviews from the medical community. The American Medical Association (AMA) ethics council originally discouraged doctors from selling vitamins and other health-related, nonprescription products from their offices. The AMA changed its statement to include recommendations for those providers who chose to sell products for profit from their offices (*www.ama-assn.org*). The AMA's recommendations include the following:

- Make sure any claims you make about the product are scientifically valid and are backed up by peer-reviewed literature and other unbiased scientific sources.
- Disclose your financial interest in any product you sell.
- Avoid monopolistic arrangements that hold patients captive. Encourage manufacturers to make it available through other channels, such as pharmacies, so that patients have a choice.

There are strong opinions supporting both sides of the issue of ethics and the sales of products through health care providers' offices. Providers are not

| Figure 15–1 | Office Procedures to Consider |

Mark the procedures you may want to master and then add to your practice:

	Yes	No	Maybe
12-Lead ECG			
Acupuncture			
Age spot removal			
Allergy evaluation and testing			
Anesthesia, topical and local			
Anoscopy			
Arthrocentesis			
Auricular hematoma evacuation			
Botox injections			
Breast biopsy			
Chalazion and hordeolum treatment			
Chest tube insertion			
Circumcision			
Collagen injections			
Colonoscopy			
Colposcopy			
Condyloma acuminata removal			
Corneal abrasion			
Cryotherapy of cervical lesions			
Debriding wounds and burns			
Defibrillation			
Diaphragm fitting			
Dislocation reduction			
Drainage of hematomas			
Ear piercing			
Endometrial biopsy			
Endotracheal intubation			
Eye trauma stabilization			
Facial chemical peels			
Flexible nasolaryngoscopy			
Flexible sigmoidoscopy			
Flu shots			
Fracture care			
Fracture immobilization			
Gastric lavage			
Hair removal			
Hypnosis			
I & D of Bartholin's cysts			
I & D of wounds			

[Continued]

Figure 15–1   **Office Procedures to Consider**   *[Continued]*

Incontinence resolution			
Infertility resolution			
Insertion of arterial, central venous, and pulmonary artery lines			
Impotence resolution			
Internal electronic fetal monitoring			
Intra-articular injection			
IUD insertion and removal			
Joint injection			
Lasers			
LEEP/LETZ/LOOP			
Lip augmentation			
Lumbar puncture			
Microdermabrasion			
Nasal packing			
Norplant insertion and removal			
Osteoporosis screening			
Paracentesis			
Pessary insertion			
Pulmonary function tests			
Radiograph interpretation			
Removal of foreign bodies			
Remove cerumen impaction			
Removing nails, skin tags, and cysts			
Retail cosmetic application			
Sclerotherapy			
Skin care			
Skin lesion biopsies and removal			
Soft tissue aspiration			
Splinting			
Suprapubic bladder aspiration			
Tattoo removal			
Thoracentesis			
Thrombosed hemorrhoid removal			
Tissue fillers			
Topical hemostasis			
Transcutaneous electrical nerve stimulation			
Trigger point injection			
Tympanometry			
Ultrasound			
Urea breath test			
Ureteral dilation			
Weight loss programs			
Wood's light examination			
Wound suturing and stapling			

only selling nutritional supplements and cosmetic creams, but many are also recruiting patients to join their multilevel marketing businesses! Be careful; there is a big difference between helping your patients by supplying scientifically tested supplements to selling non–health care related items. Some of the manufacturers of nutritional supplements include Amway, Rexall, NuSkin, Wellness International, and Interior Design Nutritionals.

If you are going to add product sales to your practice, try to find items that relate to your area of practice and will benefit your patient base—for example, pregnancy calendars, vitamins, cosmetics, skin lotions, anti-aging products, books, prostheses, wigs, weight loss programs, splints, and supports. Be sure to educate your staff on any new services or products your practice provides. Many times the patients will ask questions and your staff should be prepared with correct information. Your staff can also help promote these new services or products.

There are liability issues with the sales of vitamins and supplements to your patients. You may be held liable if you recommend products to treat conditions you are not trained to treat. Also, if you choose to treat a condition with a supplement over traditional medical treatment, you may be accused of malpractice. There is a good chance that your liability insurance coverage does not include nutritional supplement and vitamin sales—that is something to investigate.

Be sure to check with your accountant regarding state sales tax if you decide to sell products from your office. You do not want to incur costly tax problems. Selling products from your practice may enhance your bottom line significantly. However, do not ruin your reputation by becoming a salesman during your exams. You can let the patients know that the products are available—but don't push. A good rule to follow is not to recommend anything to your patients that you would not recommend for a family member in the same situation.

CLINICAL RESEARCH

Nurses have played an integral role in research throughout the years. Nurses serve as primary investigators, subinvestigators, or co-investigators for many different agencies researching clinical problems. Nurse researchers work along with or under the supervision of a principal investigator. Some nurses run the clinical trials, and many nurses are involved in research in collecting data, specimens, and communicating with the test subjects.

There are very strict regulations governing clinical research designed to protect the participants. As a nurse researcher, you must balance quality care with advancing medical knowledge. Take the time to learn all of the rules, regulations, and issues relating to research. All research with humans requires an informed consent. Study the research protocol so you know how the trial is being conducted and what is required of you.

Participating in clinical trials has been quite profitable for many independent health care providers. Contract research organizations (CROs) are charged with locating investigation sites, writing study protocols, and getting products tested. Your first step may be to locate a CRO that works within your specialty. To locate a local CRO, you can sometimes find them advertising in the newspapers for patients or even in the Yellow Pages. Online you can find information on studies being conducted by the National Institutes of Health at *www.clinicalstudies.info.nih.gov/*. The Clinical Research Investigator Registry can connect you to research companies by your specialty area at *www.criregistry.com*. Teragenix, in Ft. Lauderdale, Florida, at *www.teragenix.com* is always interested in adding providers to its database for possible future participation in research studies. Another great Website is *www.ahrq.gov* for the Agency for Healthcare Research and Quality.

Your extent of involvement in the research area varies with each study. Your role may be as small as identifying potential patients and recommending them to the study coordinators, or your role may be much more involved. Depending on the design of the study, you may have to see the patient several times and conduct several interviews, collect samples, and assess the patient.

If you have any questions regarding the ethics of a research project that you are involved with, it is your responsibility to ask questions. Ethical obligations in clinical research encompass supporting scientific thoroughness and social responsibility while protecting the subject's welfare and rights. The American Nurses Association has published an excellent resource, titled *Ethical Guidelines in the Conduct, Dissemination, and Implementation of Nursing Research* (*www.nursebooks.org*). Even if you have little or no experience in research you may be able to become involved in research and increase your revenues.

ADDING ANOTHER PROVIDER TO YOUR PRACTICE

When you bring another provider into your office, it will change the dynamics of your office environment. That may be a good thing or a not such a good thing. Whether you have another provider buy into your practice or you hire the provider to work for you, things will be different. You cannot control the other provider's practice or decisions.

Hiring another provider to help increase revenues is a great idea if your patient base can support it. You may just need to hire someone to cover your practice when you are out of town. If you are hiring a provider, follow the same procedure you follow when hiring your employees. Keep a copy of their curriculum vitae (or resume), protocol, and licensure on site. If the other provider has liability insurance, you should have a copy of the policy. Unless the provider works for you as a subcontractor, you pay him or her the same way you pay your other employees, taking out the appropriate taxes. Check with your accountant to ensure that you are following the state and federal laws.

Another option is to sell a portion of your practice to another provider. The transaction can cost a good bit of money and it also involves a good bit of risk for you. You should expect a substantial financial return. This is often done with large groups of providers, allowing them to "buy into the practice." This gives the provider more incentive to help build the practice and to make the practice more profitable.

Why would you consider selling a portion of your practice? Maybe you are feeling burned out and need some relief. Do your patients have to wait several weeks to schedule an appointment with you? Maybe you would like to change the focus of your practice and you need some help maintaining your current patient load. This is a big decision that should not be taken lightly. Once again, try to picture the worst case scenario before you make this decision.

Of course, an attorney would be necessary to complete this sale. To save money, try to think through every aspect of the sale so that when you get to the attorney you have the majority of the issues worked out. Is the financial gain worth the major changes a sale would bring? Is there enough work at your office to keep your new recruit busy? Will you need to increase your advertising significantly? Will the new practitioner bring his or her own patient base?

COMPLEMENTARY AND ALTERNATIVE THERAPIES

Studies suggest that between 30% and 50% of the adult population uses some form of complementary or alternative medicine to treat or prevent a variety of health problems. If you are interested in learning more about complementary and alternative medicine, a comprehensive resource is *Best Practices in Complementary and Alternative Medicine* by Lynda Freeman.

If you are considering including these therapies, you should first explore the issues of reimbursement. Some of these treatments are not covered by insurance, and many patients are more than willing to pay cash. However, many complementary and alternative therapies *are* covered by insurance. The billing reference book *The CAM (Complementary and Alternative Medicine) & Nursing Coding Manual* is very helpful. If these types of therapies are of interest and you are trained to prescribe them, this could be a nice way to increase your revenues as well as satisfy your patients.

SUGGESTIONS AND TIPS FROM WOMEN'S HEALTH WATCH, INC.

■ If you are interested in bringing in another provider to share your space, network with other professionals. If there is a medical newspaper or magazine for your area, you may want to place an advertisement. Word of mouth is usually the best way to find someone to share your space.

- Before you submit any articles or written material, have a friend, colleague, or family members read through the piece. They may see grammar or spelling errors that you have missed.

- Teaching has many benefits other than the obvious. Students may eventually become patients, students and faculty may refer patients to your practice, and students may be potential future employees for your practice.

- If you are adding new services and products to your practice, you need to market them to get the word out. You may want to consult a specialist in medical marketing or run your proposed marketing materials or plans by a few of your colleagues. An error in this area has the potential to damage your image.

PERSONAL ANECDOTES

- Since I was working two half-days per week for my physician of protocol, my office was available for other providers to use during that time. I rented an exam room to an occupational therapist and brought in extra income for my practice.

- Over the years, many of my patients were involved in research studies. We had a super arrangement with Millennium Biotech (which is now Teragenix) to supply blood products from patients with certain characteristics to researchers. This participation significantly increased our revenues and we were able to reward the patients involved in the studies with extra samples and discounts.

Resources

American Association of Legal Nurse Consultants: *www.aalnc.org.*
American Nurses Association: Ethical Guidelines in the Conduct, Dissemination, and Implementation of Nursing Research: *www.nursebooks.org.*
American Nurses Publishing, 600 Maryland Avenue, Southwest, Suite 100, West Washington, DC 20024-2571: *www.nursesbooks.org* or 202-651-7000.
American Medical Association: *www.ama-assn.org.*
Astin, J, Marie, A, Pelletier, KR, Hansen, E, and Haskell, WL: A review of the incorporation of complementary and alternative medicine by mainstream physicians. JAMA [online, November 23, 1998]: *http://archinte.ama-assn.org/issues/v158n21/abs/ira80434.html.*
Billing reference: Procedural codes, definitions for complementary and alternative medicine and nursing. Albany, NY: Delmar Publishing, 2001.
Bradigan, PS, Powell, CA, and Van Brimmer, B: Writer's guide to nursing and allied health journals. Washington, DC: American Nurses Publishing, 1998.
CAM & Nursing Coding Manual, 1st ed. Albany: Delmar Publishing, 2001.
Carnegie, D: How to develop self-confidence and influence people by public speaking. New York: Carnegie and Associates, 1999.

Carnegie, D: The quick and easy way to effective speaking. New York: Dale Carnegie and Associates, 1990.

Carter, MA: Procedures for nurse practitioners. Des Moines: Springhouse, 2001.

Clinical Research Investigator Registry: *www.criregistry.com*.

Colyar, MR, and Ehardt, CR: Ambulatory care procedures for the nurse practitioner. Philadelphia: FA Davis, 1999.

Dale Carnegie Courses: *www.westegg.com*.

Davis, KM., Clark D, and Koch, KE: Physician marketing of nutritional supplements. JAMA [online, September 16, 1998]: *http://www.jama.ama.-assn.org/issues/ v280nll/ffull/jlt0916-6.html*.

Emanuel, EJ, Wendler, D, and Grady, C: What makes clinical research ethical? JAMA [online, May 24, 2000]: *http://www.jama.ama-assn.rog/issues/ v283n20/abs/jsc90374.html*.

FA Davis Company, 1915 Arch Street, Philadelphia, PA 19103: *www.fadavis.com* or 1-800-523-4049.

Finger, AL: Want to boost revenue? Mount a collection campaign. Medical Economics [online, March 19, 2001] 6,68: *http://www.me.pdr.net*.

Forster, J: Memo from the editor: The money you're missing out on. Medical Economics [online, February 19, 2001] 4,7: *http://www.me.pdr.net/ me/psrecord.htm*.

Freeman, LW: Best practices in complementary and alternative medicine. Gaithersburg, MD: Aspen Publishers, 2001.

Fulton, L: Directory of small press and magazine editors & publishers, 30th ed. New York: Dustbooks, 2001.

Gianelli, DM: Ethics council revisits office-based product sales. American Medical News [online, June 7, 1999]: *http://www.ama-assn.org/sci-pubs/ amnesw/pick_99/anna0607.htm*.

Gianelli, DM: Physicians as sales reps? American Medical News [online, November 24, 1997]: *http://www.ama-assn.org/sci-pubs/amnews/pick1124.htm*.

Grady, C: Clinical research: The power of the nurse. Am J Nursing 101(9):11, 2001.

Gunn, SJ: Natural healing: Alternative, complementary resources for total health. Newberg, OR: Bookpartners, Inc, 1999.

Jiorle, L: Trading stethoscopes for law books. Clinician News 17:4–5, 2001.

Kaplan College: *www.kaplancollege.edu/LN* or 1-800-669-2555.

Karigan, M: Ethics in clinical research. American Journal of Nursing, 101(9):26–31, 2001.

Kenner, C, and Walden, M: Grant writing tips for nurses and other health professionals. Washington, DC: American Nurses Publishing, 2001.

Medical-Legal Consulting Institute, PMB 632, 2476 Bolsover Street, Houston, TX 77005: *www.legalnurse.com*. or 1-800-880-0944.

Miller, SK: Performing clinical procedures. Patient Care for the Nurse Practitioner 12:70–71, 2000.

National Institutes of Health: *www.clinicalstudies.info.nih.gov/*.

NCLEX: *www.ncsbn.org* or 312-787-6555 extension 496.

National Procedures Institute: *www.NPInstitute* or 1-800-462-2492.

Physician's Payment Update (February 2001): *http://www.ahcpub.com/online.html*.

PDR for herbal medicines: Dallas: Physicians' Drug Reference, 1998.

Restrepo, A, Davitt, C, and Thompson, S: House calls: Is there an APN in the house? J Am Acad Nurse Pract 13(12):560–564, 2001.

Rozaskis, LE: The complete idiot's guide to public speaking. New York: Alpha Books, 1999.

Small Business Association (SBA): *www.sba.gov*.

Speak Easy Seminars: *www.speakeasy.net*.

Speech Tips: *www.speechtips.com*.

Teragenix: *www.teragenix.com*.

Toastmasters International: *www.toastmasters.org*.

Vista Writer's Guide: *www.vistameded.com* or 209-476-8673.

Waldrop, JB: Getting back to basics. Clin Advisor 12:100, 2000.

Wilder, C, and Fine, D: Point, click and wow!! A quick guide to brilliant laptop presentations. New York: Pfeiffer and Company, 1996.

Wilder, C: Slides that win and presentation points [CD-ROM]. Boston: Wilder, 2001.

Wilder, C: Presentations *www.wilderpresentations.com* or 617-524-7172.

Wilder, L: 7 Steps to fearless speaking. New York: John Wiley and Sons, 1999.

Zaslove, MO: The successful physician: A productivity handbook for practitioners. Gaithersburg, MD: Aspen Publications, 1998.

NOTES

Chapter 16

Technologies Used in Practice: Do I Really Need to Buy New Stuff?

" We are told never to cross a bridge until we come to it, but this world is owned by men who have "crossed bridges" in their imagination far ahead of the crowd "

Speakers Library

As you know, technology changes so rapidly, it is difficult to keep up. The new technologies can greatly enhance your practice—but they do come at a price. You can reduce time and energy previously spent doing things by hand. Just think of how much easier it is to produce a letter on your computer compared to a manual typewriter. This chapter explores the technologies and may give you some ideas that may increase your efficiency level and leave you with more time for your patients.

COMPUTERS

The days of running a medical practice with just a pegboard and a telephone are over. Insurance companies are now demanding electronic filing of claims, which requires a computer. A computer for your office is a necessity that, in the long run, will increase your profits. It doesn't have to be the top of the line or super expensive. If you are starting a solo practice from scratch, a personal computer will be sufficient for your first few years. The software you install on your computer will dictate the choice of the hardware required. Be sure to secure accessibility to technical support for both the computer and the software programs. If a problem arises, it is nice to know that you have access to help. If you are purchasing a new computer, you may want to consider buying the computer and your software from the same source, so one can't blame the other if there is a problem.

Computers can be purchased from a variety of sources. You can shop at the big retailers in your area, shop online, or purchase from a local vendor. You may be able to get the best price from the big retailer, whereas the local vendor may be able to give you more prompt and personalized service.

When purchasing a computer, compare all the computers in your price range. Try to get the most advanced system for your money. If you have friends or family members who are computer savvy, enlist their help in the selection process. A good rule is to try to buy one step behind the newest technology. The newest technology is always the most expensive. Avoid purchasing a used computer system. You may be buying a lot of headaches with a used computer. Shop around, just as you would for a new car. See Figure 16–1 for a computer buying checklist.

The processor is basically the brain of the computer. It controls all of the actions within the computer. This is the most important component to consider when purchasing your new computer. Get the most processor for your money. The processor speed is basically how fast the computer runs. The higher the megahertz, the faster your computer will run. New and faster processors are always being developed. As the faster processors become available, the slower processors are phased out.

The RAM (random access memory) is commonly referred to as the memory of the computer. This memory is measured in megabytes (MB). This is the second most important item to consider in your purchasing process. The RAM is the temporary storage area for the computer while it is working. The more RAM you have, the faster the computer can perform the tasks requested. The more RAM, the better. This is an area that can be upgraded later if necessary.

The cache is another type of memory, which is similar to the RAM. The computer uses the cache to move data between the RAM and the processor. Again—more is better! The motherboard is the circuit board where all the components are connected. The processor, RAM chips, and cache all plug into the motherboard. The more plug-in slots that the motherboard contains, the better. Basically, the main considerations in a motherboard for you to consider are the number of expansion slots and the number of RAM slots.

The computer case type you decide on really just depends on your desk layout. Some people prefer having the tower on the floor whereas others like it to be more accessible on their desk surface. One does not work better than the other; it is really just what fits your office best.

The hard drive is where most of your programs that you install will be stored. This important part of the computer cannot be seen from the outside. The more programs you install, the more hard drive space you will need. Again, more is better.

There are several different ways to store the data you put into your computer. The traditional way is to use a floppy disk drive. The floppy disk drive provides an easy way to save and transport files between computers.

Most computers come with a CD-ROM drive as a standard component. Most computer programs now come on CDs. The CD-ROM drives come in several different speeds. The faster the CD-ROM drive; the better. CD writers are

| **Figure 16–1** | **Computer Buying Checklist** |

	Your Preference	Computer #1	Computer #2	Computer #3
Processor type				
Processor speed				
RAM (Memory)				
Cache				
Motherboard				
Case (tower or desktop)				
Hard drive capacity (GB)				
CD-ROM				
Tape, zip, or CD backup system				
Mouse				
Keyboard				
Monitor				
Video card				
Printer				
Modem				
Toll-free technical support				
Price				

Copyright © 2003, F.A. Davis Company

now available that allow you to write (or copy) information onto a CD. This may be a good solution to data storage problems.

A tape backup drive is mainly used for backing up (or saving) the files that are on your hard drive. The tapes can hold a lot of information. The tape backup is an excellent tool for saving your medical program and financial data. This should be backed up weekly, if not daily. One tape should be taken off the premises in case of fire or theft. In the event of computer failure, theft, or the purchase of a new computer, the tape backup will enable your computer technician to restore your files and have your new computer up and running quickly.

A zip drive is removable storage similar to the floppy drive. This is a good alternative to the tape backup if you don't have a lot of data to back up. For a medical practice, the tape would be your best bet, unless you master the CD writer.

The mouse is a very important device for your new computer. The mouse is good for pointing to and moving objects on the screen. There are several variations to the mouse—it is basically the preference of the user that will guide you with this purchase. Alternatives to the mouse include the touch pad, trackball and touch screen.

The differences in keyboards are minimal. The descriptors of the different keyboards usually center around how many keys are on the keyboards. Ergonomic keyboards are shaped to be easier on the user's wrists.

Several different sizes of monitors are available. Again, this is an area where personal preference and costs are the deciding factors. The cost of the monitor may not be included in the cost of the computer system, so be sure to check for the monitor in the system package.

The video card is the component of the computer that sends images to the computer monitor. Video cards are also referred to as video accelerators. The video card usually contains a memory chip that will allow the computer to load images quickly.

A good quality printer is a worthwhile investment. There are three different types of printers available: dot matrix (outdated), ink-jet or bubble-jet, and laser printer. A laser printer is optimal, but is really not necessary for your practice. If the ink-jet or bubble-jet is more fitting to your budget, it should produce a nicely printed product. Some printers also function as a fax, copier, and scanner. Shop around for what is appropriate for you.

A modem is required if you want to access the Internet through your computer. The modem also allows you to send and receive faxes with your computer. Most computers include the modem as a standard component. The modem allows your computer to communicate with other computers through your telephone line. The higher speed modem produces faster transmission of data. Before you purchase a modem, check your billing software for the recommended speed. Newer, faster modems may not be compatible for transferring data with slower systems.

Don't forget to protect your new computer with a surge protector! A surge protector is an inexpensive way to protect against power spikes. If there is a big thunderstorm on the way, your best protection is to unplug your system and the telephone line to your modem. Be sure your office insurance policy covers your computers for theft and storm damage.

When choosing a medical software program, ask other providers what programs they use. Find a program that is easy to use and that comes with great technical support. If the software program is not easy to learn and use, you may be wasting a lot of your staff's time. Get plenty of training for your staff. It is a lot more efficient to learn as much as possible in the beginning, rather than on the go. You should learn the programs as well. Learn how to access information without assistance. Learn all aspects of the program so you can get your full value out of the program. Ask about the program's schedule and costs of upgrades. Most medical software programs have yearly upgrades. The cost may seem high, but it may be worth your money to have the most current version of your program. It is more important to secure good training and ongoing support than to get a bargain on your equipment and software.

THE INTERNET

The Internet has so much to offer health care providers. It is great for researching the latest treatment recommendations. Patient information handouts and journal articles can be easily accessed on the Internet. The Internet has become a professional tool for accessing many different types of information as well as for communicating with other facilities and providers.

Start an address book of sites that are appropriate for your practice. Many journal articles will identify sites that may be of interest to you. Some sites related to clinical practice include:

- Centers for Disease Control and Prevention: *www.cdc.gov*
- National Library of Medicine's Internet Grateful Med and PubMed: *www.ncbi.nlm.nih.gov/pubmed*
- Medscape: *www.medscape.com*
- Physician's Desk Reference: *www.pdr.net*
- New England Journal of Medicine: *www.nejm.org*
- The Lancet: *www.thelancet.com*
- British Medical Journal: *www.mj.com*
- NPLinx: *www.NPLinx.com*

TELEMEDICINE

Telemedicine (also called telehealth or e-health) refers to health care provided through cables and cyberspace. Telemedicine is impacting health care providers, institutions, pharmaceutical companies, the medical equipment industry, and patients. Health care systems are coordinating patient data with the goal of keeping paperless records. Computer passwords are being replaced with sophisticated technology to achieve a more secure system of accessing information, such as evaluating one's iris, voice, or fingerprints.

Providers and institutions are purchasing supplies on the Internet and are enjoying significant savings. Managed care and insurance companies are allowing online access to personal health insurance information and provider authorizations. Health care providers, institutions, and health plans are sponsoring Websites. Hospitals are using the Internet for claims and prescription handling, along with provider credentialing and directories.

Health care providers are more accessible to their patients by using e-mail. Patients are accessing the Internet for health information. In outlying areas where specialists are scarce, some have taken to using video conferencing to diagnose and treat their patients. Many are concerned about licensing issues when crossing state lines. This is an area to watch. We will see tremendous growth in telemedicine and it may present some great opportunities for entrepreneurial nurse practitioners!

ELECTRONIC MEDICAL RECORDS SYSTEMS

Electronic medical records (EMR) systems are the future for managing medical records. Many practices have already converted to EMR systems. Implementing these systems can be costly, and it may be best to wait until your practice is established for a few years before making the investment. It is estimated that the learning curve (and a reduction of productivity) can take approximately 3 to 6 months when implementing the new EMR system. Some of the benefits of the EMR systems include:

- Less work for support staff (eventually, less staff required)
- No charts to pull before the patient's arrival
- Lab results available immediately
- Time saved with documentation
- Time saved looking through old records

Current users of the EMR systems state that the EMR is a valuable tool to enhance productivity, income, quality, and patient acceptance.[1] Ask other providers about EMR systems if you are interested. Another provider's input could be valuable in this situation. Ask to go to the other provider's office and watch them actually use the EMR system, then speak with the EMR system representative.

Features to look for when evaluating EMR systems include:

- Billing capabilities with coding information
- Ability to print a current charge slip at the end of a visit
- Ability to handle multiple insurers for each patient
- Ability to batch entries
- Open item posting that tracks charges by each item
- Easy access for entering new patient information
- Ability to produce recalls and reminders for patient visits
- Report sequencing to break down overdue bills by payer, or even by patient
- Ability to evaluate productivity by level of visits
- Ability to produce summary sheets

Some EMR systems are integrated with voice recognition technology, meaning that you can dictate directly into your computer. ChartLogic by Task Technologies is one such program. Again, do your homework and know what you want from the EMR system before you commit to installation.

WEBSITE DEVELOPMENT

Do you need a Website for your practice? Of course, you can start without one and develop your site once your practice is up and running. Or, you can develop a site from the start with the thought that the extra exposure a Website can give your practice will certainly increase your revenues. The Internet is an attractive opportunity for nurse practitioners wanting to build or increase their patient base. Many people search for providers on the Internet. Many patients are not only looking for providers with Websites, but they also want to have additional information on the provider, such as education, experience, hours, specialty, and location before they commit to scheduling an appointment.

Some entrepreneurs feel that a good Website is a marketing necessity. If you are going to proceed with creating a Website for your practice, you must make a plan. First, write out all the important information you think would be beneficial for a potential patient to know about you and your practice. Some things you may want to include in your site may be:

- Your photograph
- Brief biography (including licenses and certifications)
- Office location with a map
- Office hours
- Hospital affiliations

- Insurance/HMO programs
- Special procedures
- Contact information (address, telephone, fax, e-mail)
- Emergency contact information
- Photographs of your office
- Links to appropriate health information Websites
- Anything else that you think would be interesting to a prospective patient

Two common mistakes that Internet newcomers make are to invest a lot of money in an elaborate design and to assume that Website traffic will automatically appear. You have to budget in the ongoing expense of making continuous updates with major search engines to ensure that rankings remain high.

There is the cost of updating the contents and maintaining the site. The goal is to keep your Website online, up-to-date, and easily found for a reasonable fee. You want your site to be quick loading and search engine friendly. Again, if you have a friend or family members who have experience in this area, you may benefit from their input. There are many Web design and maintenance businesses eager for new clients. Be smart and shop around. Know what you are getting for your money. Also, put on your calendar a reminder to log onto your site on a regular basis and examine the content. Communicate with your Web master any changes you would like to see implemented. An Internet presence shows your practice is on the cutting edge of the many changes in health care. A Website may also enhance your image in the medical community and demonstrate that your profession is advancing as a leader in health care, not as a follower.

E-MAIL COMMUNICATION WITH YOUR PATIENTS

Many providers are encouraging their patients to contact them through e-mail. This communication is sometimes called "e-connectivity," and it links providers with patients. E-mail offers the patient another avenue in reaching their providers. E-mail communication is often faster and more accurate than leaving telephone messages. You can also communicate easier with your patient's family members who may be out of state. E-mail enhances the medical record in that you can produce a printed copy of your communication. Patients may feel more comfortable discussing personal and sensitive issues by e-mail. They may also have the feeling that they are not "bothering" the provider by interrupting their schedule for a telephone call. The provider can set a time in the daily schedule to check and respond to e-mail. By using e-mail for some patient communication, you can reduce the telephone calls to your office and the "telephone tag" that usually follows.

If you do decide to communicate with your patients by e-mail, you must make it very clear to them that this communication method is not for emergencies. Just as you don't diagnose over the telephone, do not diagnose online. You can encourage your patients to call for an appointment and instruct them on what they can do in the meantime. There are some legal issues and privacy matters you should know before corresponding this way. A simple signed consent form may help defend you in the event of a lawsuit. You should set some guidelines for your e-mail communication. You may want to develop a form for your patients to fill out during their first visit inquiring whether they would like to be able to communicate with their provider online. Outline the limitations of e-mail communication as well as the potential risks. List out the rules you have developed, such as to call the office for emergencies or to discuss time-sensitive issues or personal information, or if your response is delayed. Have the patient include his or her name in the subject line, and be concise.

When communicating by e-mail, use the appropriate form, content, and tone. It is easy to lapse into a more casual line of conversation, but that may not be appropriate. Try to avoid irony, sarcasm, humor, and harsh criticisms. E-mail communication can be used best to convey prescription refill requests, to receive test results, to answer questions, to give advice, to schedule appointments, to reply to requests for health information, and to clarify treatment plans. E-mail communications should be printed and included in the patient's chart.

Having the ability to respond to e-mail from your patients regarding their concerns and having the capability to attach educational material about their concerns can be can be very helpful and appreciated. You can create your own virtual library by writing your own patient handouts. There are also patient handouts available on CD-ROM from the American Academy of Family Physicians at *www.familydoctor.org*. When purchasing the book *Griffith's Instructions for Patients*, a CD-ROM with patient handouts is included.

Your e-mail service should allow you to develop an address book, make copies of your messages, and sign the message. There is also a receipt feature that will notify you when the recipient receives the e-mail. A dedicated telephone line for your fax and computer will help keep your patient telephone lines free. More detailed information is included in the *Guidelines for the Clinical Use of Electronic Mail with Patients* by Drs. Beverly Kane and Daniel Sands.

ProMinders is a Web-based notification system that enables you to connect with patients by sending them messages via e-mail, fax, or telephone in your own voice and in any language. More information is available at *www.prominders.com*.

MAINTAINING PATIENT PRIVACY

Maintaining patient privacy has been an objective that has been drilled into our brains since we first started in our basic nursing programs. The importance of not talking about our patients outside the classroom was stressed over and over. Since the passage of the Healthcare Insurance Portability and Accountability Act of 1996 (HIPAA) even more emphasis will be placed on health care professionals and patient privacy. HIPAA is now the standard for confidentiality throughout the country. Penalties for inappropriate disclosure of patient information begin at $50,000 and 1 year in jail—this is a strong incentive to comply with HIPAA.

The HIPAA rule covers all medical records and other health information that is stored or communicated electronically, on paper, or orally. Patients have significant rights under this rule regarding how their health information is used.

The HIPAA rules can be found at *http://aspe.hhs.gov/admnsimp/ final/txfin00.htm*. You should print out this rule, read it, and teach your employees the rules. Would you like a $50,000 fine for a simple error made by your employee that could have been prevented? It could happen! Learn the rules and follow them.

Assign all employees computer passwords to enter your medical data program. If you are using e-mail to communicate with your patients regarding sensitive topics, you should really install an encryption system. And most importantly, you must train your employees about the importance of protecting the patient's confidentiality.

SUGGESTIONS AND TIPS FROM WOMEN'S HEALTH WATCH, INC.

- When upgrading the computer, we did not check with the representative from our Medicaid billing office. We bought the newest and fastest modem available. Three days later we were paying to have it removed and replaced with our old modem. The new modem was too fast for the old billing program that Medicaid used.

- Our computer was hit three different times by lightning. It always happened during off hours. We believe the power surge came through the telephone line and fried the motherboard. Luckily, all three times the office insurance covered the replacement costs. However, we did have down time when we were unable to access our patient's billing information.

- We had a tape drive installed and performed regular backups. That really paid off after the lightning strikes to our computer. We were able to have our new computer up and running within about 3 days after the thunderstorm.

PERSONAL ANECDOTES

1. I resisted developing a Website for the practice for many years. I wish I had designed it early on. I didn't realize how many people depend on the Internet instead of the telephone book!

2. I did have a potential patient contact me through my e-mail. She is very shy and had a few questions she needed answered before she could schedule an appointment. I answered her questions and even scheduled her appointment via e-mail. Over time, she became one of my favorite patients!

Resources

American Academy of Family Physicians: Patient education handouts: *www.familydoctor.org.*

Bauer, J, and Ringel, M: Telemedicine and the reinvention of healthcare: The seventh revolution in medicine. New York: McGraw-Hill, 1999.

Carter, JH: Electronic medical records: A guide for clinicians and administrators. Philadelphia: American College of Physicians, 2001.

ChartLogic, Task Technologies: 888-337-4441.

Computer purchasing information, International Computer Negotiations: *www.dobetterdeals.com.*

Delta, GB, and Matsuura, JH: Law of the Internet. New York: Aspen, 1997.

Griffith's Instructions for Patients: Philadelphia: WB Saunders, 1998.

Kane, B, and Sands, DZ: (January-February, 1998). Guidelines for the clinical use of electronic mail with patients. Journal of the American Medical Informatics Association [online, January-February 1998]: *http://www.amia.org/pubs/pospaper/positio2.htm* or 1-800-819-2334, document #406.

Knopper, M: The telemedicine takeoff: Is this long-distance technology a short distance away? Clinician News 24:1–23, 2001.

Kraft, S, and Rehm, S: How to select a computer system for a family physician's office, Kansas City, MO: American Academy of Family Physicians, 1998.

Leawood, KS: American Academy of Family Physicians: *www.aafp.org.*

Lippman, H: Re-engineering your practice: Never lose a chart again. Medical Economics Magazine [online, July 24, 2000], 3: *http://www.pdr.net/memag/public.htm?path=docs/article3.html.*

Lowes, R: Switching from paper to computerized charts. Medical Economics Magazine [online, May 24, 1999], 24: *http://www.pdr.net/memag/static.htm?path=docs/052499/article2.html.*

Lowes, R: Why that computer "bargain" may be anything but. Medical Economics Magazine [online, November 22, 1999] 22,63: *http://www.me.pdr.net/me/prescord.htm.*

Mangan, D: Save time and please patients with e-mail. Medical Economics Magazine [online, July 12, 1999] 12: *http://www.pdr.net/memag/public.htm?path=docs/071299/article2.html.*

Medical Software Reviews Newsletter: *www.healthcarecomputing.com.*

Pearson, L: E-health and HIPAA: Important emerging issues affecting our practice. The Nurse Practitioner 26(April):10–14, 2001.

Sands, DZ: Guidelines for the use of patient centered e-mail. Massachusetts Health Data Consortium [online, 1999]: *http://www.mahealthdata.org.* or call 781-890-6040.

Simpson, K: When communication starts to click. The Clinical Advisor 35(April):36, 2001.

Skepple, AT: Move your practice online. Advance for Nurse Practitioners 4(December):16, 2000.

Sterling, R: Guide to medical practice software. New York: Harcourt Professional Publishing, 1999: *www.hbpp.com* or 1-800-831-7799.

Tumulo, J: You've got mail! Advance for Nurse Practitioners 43(February):86–91, 2001.

Reference

1. Basch, P: Electronic records—I can't live without 'em. Medical Economics Magazine [online, December 6, 1999] 14: *http://me.pdr.net/me/psrecord.htm? NS_doc_offset= 1&NS_doc_returned=12&NS.*

NOTES

Selling Your Practice

Chapter 17

Selling the Practice: How Do I?

" Success has always been easy to measure. It is the distance between one's origins and one's final achievement "

Michael Korda

When you are designing and building your new practice, selling your practice is probably the last thing you are thinking about. It should not be. It is often said that the first thing you should plan for when you start a business is the day you will sell it. When you were writing your business plan, you may have been a bit stumped when you reached the section labeled "exit plan." The exit plan is basically the section where you explore how you want to leave your practice. You should think about your future and your practice before you are in the position in which you need or want to sell your practice. Design the practice so it has the maximum value (with or without you). You should design your practice in a way that will bring you the best return on your investment. Thinking about selling your practice before you are ready to sell may help prepare you for this important transaction.

There are many different scenarios that may lead you to selling the practice you have designed and built. You may think you will be enjoying your practice forever, but circumstances change and unforeseen events may lead you to sell. Some reasons for selling include retirement, boredom, illness, relocation, partner disputes, and financial disappointment. Or, possibly, you may not enjoy being a business owner. If life leads you to this point, you should feel good that you have built something of value. Instead of "paying rent" (working for others) you have "built a house" (your practice) that is worth some money.

Before you put your practice on the market, establish your goals and strategies for the upcoming sale. By completing this activity, you will be better prepared to attain your goals by implementing the strategies you have decided upon. Some questions that may help you set your goals and design your strategies include:

- What are your main reasons for selling your practice?
- What would you like to personally gain from the sale?
- How do you see your practice after the sale?
- Are you willing to sell the name of your practice?
- Are there specific characteristics you require in a buyer?
- Do you want to stay affiliated with your practice after the sale? Just during the transition or indefinitely?
- What financial terms are you ready to accept? Must it be all cash? Will you finance a portion of the sale if you can get a higher price?
- If you own the office building, do you want to sell it or lease it?

Some of the things that you will also need to think about include preparing your practice for sale and finding a viable buyer. You will need to prepare documents and also prepare the practice to be seen in its best light. Make sure that your practice is presentable. A business that is clean with a current inventory and with equipment in good working order sells the fastest. Finding a buyer may take some creative thinking and lots of networking. Again, try to enjoy the learning process and also enjoy the selling process.

Some tips to help you prepare your practice to bring you the best sale price include:

- Start your practice with the thought that you will eventually be selling it.
- Before you are faced with the task, think about how and when would be ideal to sell your practice.
- Continuously provide the best possible services and products so you build the biggest and best business possible.
- Maintain your professional business image that you have created. Make an effort to make your practice appear even more professional and successful than it really is.
- Consult with your legal counsel to ensure your practice is structured properly for a sale.
- Allow enough time for you to adjust to selling your practice—both financially and emotionally.

You may also want to consider whom you will tell about the sale of your practice and when you will tell them. Planning is once again very important; think through the pros and cons of sharing the news with the different people associated with your practice. It may take more than a year to sell your practice and you don't want your patient base and employees to disappear because they heard you were leaving. Tell your family and close friends well before you tell anyone else about the sale. Then, hopefully, you will have their support and understanding during this stressful time. Of course, you also need to consult with your attorney and accountant. Their input can be invaluable at this stage of the game. Take notes during the conversations and provide them with any requested materials swiftly. You may also want to let them know that they can feel free to pass the word to fellow colleagues and potential buyers about your practice coming up for sale. Word of mouth can be your best marketing tool for selling your practice.

Make a list of your vendors, insurance companies, pharmaceutical companies, laboratories, telephone companies, advertising media, credit card processing company, Medicaid, Medicare, biohazardous waste company, banks, utility companies, landlord, insurance brokers, and so on (Fig. 17–1). They will need to be notified once the sale is completed.

DEFINING WHAT YOU WILL BE SELLING

The first step in preparing for the sale of your practice is actually defining what you are selling. The total number of patient charts, the fixed assets of the practice, and your goodwill are the three areas that usually help define health-care practices that are for sale.

You may want to have your staff physically count your charts or you may be able to gather this information from your computer software program. You may also want to count how many of the charts are for current patients and how many are for patients who haven't been in the office within the past 2 years.

The fixed assets are the physical items that you are offering to sell along with the patient charts. These items may include desks, telephones, computers, fax machines, exam tables, medical equipment, and much more. The fixed assets should be inventoried either by categories or by the location of the items. You should also estimate the replacement cost of each item and include it on the inventory. This will help you in assigning a total value for the fixed assets of your practice (Fig. 17–2)

When selling a practice, goodwill is defined as an intangible asset, representing the excess cost over the fixed assets and charts. Goodwill is the perceived value of the practice's name, reputation, and anticipated stream of earnings. The buyer is purchasing the good reputation and name that you have worked so hard to create and maintain.

You must confer with your legal counsel regarding the type of business structure you have established (sole proprietorship, corporation, or a limited liability company). The structure of your business will determine exactly what you are able to sell. For example, with a sole proprietorship you cannot sell the stocks but can sell the assets.

Figure 17-1 Notification of Sale Checklist.

Who (use additional paper as needed)	When	Done
Family:		
Friends:		
Attorney: Accountant: Others:		
Employees:		
Vendors:		
Banks:		
Pharmaceutical Company Representatives:		
Utility & Telephone Companies:		
Referring Providers:		
Insurance Companies:		
Medicare and Medicaid Offices:		
Patients		

| **Figure 17–2** | Sample Fixed Asset Inventory Sheet |

Women's Health Watch, Inc.
1999 OFFICE INVENTORY

Included in Sale

Reception/Entry
6 SECTIONAL CHAIRS—INDIAN COTTON $450

1 SILK TREE—7' $125

1 WICKER BASKET $5

2 MANET FRAMED POSTERS $40 EA.

1 LITERATURE RACK $50

Front Office
2 DESK CHAIRS ZENITH OFFICE SUPPLY $100 EA

1 DESK 5'×3'×3' WOOD $250

3 FILE CABINETS-2/5 DRAWER $800 EA - 1/6 DRAWER $900

1 MICROWAVE OVEN-SHARP CAROUSEL 2 $100

1 MICROWAVE STAND $50

1 COMPUTER DESK $250

1 PENTIUM 11 MMX 350 MHZ PCI BUS COMPUTER $1500

1 COMPUTER KEYBOARD KEY TRONIC $100

1 COMPUTER MONITOR TATUNG $150

1 FELLOWES COPY HOLDER $20

1 HEWLETT PACKER OFFICE JET PRINTER/FAX/COPIER $450

1 CANON PC COPIER $500

1 AVANTI REFRIGERATOR 3'×2'×2' $125

1 BROTHER ELECTRIC TYPEWRITER AX-250 $200

2 WASTE BASKETS 1—$5 1—$15

1 SET OAK DESK ACCESSORIES $20

2 SILK PLANTS IN HANGING BASKETS $25 EA

1 PLASTIC CHAIR MAT $25

1 WOODEN QUARTZ CLOCK $20

1 PROCTER SILEX COFFEE POT $15

1 CASIO ADDING MACHINE $40

1 BATTERY BACKUP TRIPP LITE $150

1 SURGE PROTECTOR ISOTEL $75

1 CREDIT CARD PROCESSING MACHINE 1-TRANZ 380—$400

1 CREDIT CARD PRINTER $250

2 GE 4 LINE/SPEAKER PHONE SYSTEM $200 EA

1 CORK BOARD 3'×2' $15

MISC OFFICE SUPPLIES $500

PATIENT CHARTS - APPROX. 3000

Not included in Sale

1 ILLUMINATED EXIT SIGN 1
EMERGENCY LIGHTING SIGN
WINDOW TREATMENTS
PERSONAL AWARDS

1 PITNEY BOWES POSTAGE
MACHINE—RENTAL
1 KIDD FIRE EXTINGUISHER
1 HUNTER CEILING FAN

[Continued]

| **Figure 17–2** | **Sample Fixed Asset Inventory Sheet** *[Continued]* |

Hallway

1 GE 4 LINE/SPEAKER PHONE SYSTEM $200

1 GI TRACT TEACHING MODEL $150

1 FRAMED BOTERO POSTER 35" × 46" $250

1 FRAMED POSTER OF FLOWERS 30" × 35" $125

1 ZEPHYRHILLS WATER COOLER—RENTAL

2 ILLUMINATED EXIT SIGNS

1 EMERGENCY LIGHTING SYSTEM

Exam Room #1

1 EXAM TABLE WITH STIRRUPS, SEVILLE 5 DRAWER $450

1 CHAIR WOOD & RUSH $50

1 ROLLING STOOL $120

1 CABINET 2 DRAWER & CUPBOARD $180

1 COLPOSCOPE WITH CAMERA $4500

1 FOOT PEDAL WASTE CAN $90

2 HEAD LIGHTS $135

1 FLOATING ARM MAGNIFIER LAMP $260

1 FRAMED NEW MEXICO POSTER—RC GORMAN $100

MISC. INSTRUMENTS AND SUPPLIES $200

1 PAPER TOWEL DISPENSER STAINLESS

1 SOAP DISPENSER

Lab Area

1 CABINET 2 DRAWER & CUPBOARD $180

1 CRYO HANDPIECE $1,000 (Tank is rented—not included)

1 STAINLESS STEEL UTILITY CART $160

1 HIGH DIRECTOR'S CHAIR $75

1 DETECTO SCALE $250

1 BEAD STERILIZER $300

1 FORMICA COUNTERTOP $200

1 HEMOCUE $250—Hgb

1 SWING ARM LAMP $12

1 LARGE WASTE BASKET METAL $25

1 HOOVER UPRIGHT VACCUM $125

5 COLPOSCOPY INSTRUMENTS $500

MISC. INSTRUMENTS AND SUPPLIES $500

1 PAPER TOWEL DISPENSER STAINLESS

1 SOAP DISPENSER

Office

1 DESK WOOD 5' × 3' $450

1 CREDENZA WOOD 1.5' × 5' $250

1 DESK CHAIR OVERSTUFFED $200

3 WOOD & RUSH CHAIRS $50 EA

1 END TABLE, WOOD $75

1 TYPING TABLE $50

1 TRACK LIGHTING UNIT

1 CEILING FAN HUNTER

PERSONAL DIPLOMAS AND AWARDS

REFERENCE BOOKS

DESK & CREDENZA CONTENTS

Figure 17–2 Sample Fixed Asset Inventory Sheet *[Continued]*

1 SILK PLANT $50

1 MICROSCOPE $500

1 BRASS LAMP/SHADE $120

1 GE 4 LINES/SPEAKER PHONE SYSTEM $200

1 COMPUTER PST 486 33 MEG $1,000

1 MONITOR SANTRON $150

1 KEYBOARD VENDEX HEADSTART $100

1 HEWLETT-PACKARD DESK JET COLOR PRINTER $400

1 SURGE PROTECTOR $20

1 METAL STEP-ON WASTE CAN $60

1 FRAMED BOTERO POSTER 3.5′ × 2.5′ $150

Patient Bathroom

1 WASTE BASKET $5

2 FRAMED PRINTS SHELLS $25 EA

Employee Bathroom

1 WASTEBASKET $5

2 4 -SHELF BOOKCASES $40 EA

1 WOOD CABINET W/MIRRORS

1 STAINLESS TOWEL DISPENSER

1 SOAP DISPENSER

Back Room

1 FILE CABINET 4 DRAWER $50

1 MICROWAVE STAND PORTABLE $50

1 ROLLING STOOL $120

1 FOOT PEDAL WASTE CAN $90

1 EMERGENCY EYE WASH UNIT $70

1 DRY ERASER BOARD 2′ × 3′ $45

1 WASTEBASKET $5

1 GE 4 LINE/SPEAKER PHONE SYSTEM $200

1 STAINLESS TOWEL DISPENSER

1 SOAP DISPENSER

1 ILLUMINATED EXIT SIGN

1 EMERGENCY LIGHTING SYSTEM

1 REFRIGERATOR—LOAN - MB

1 CENTRIFUGE—LOAN - MB

1 KIDD FIRE EXTINGUISHER

Storage Unit

1 EXAM TABLE WITH STIRRUPS $450

1 PROCTER SILEX COFFEE POT $15

* Secutity System hardware is not included

PRESENTING YOUR PRACTICE ON PAPER

You know that your practice is wonderful—now you want to convince your prospective buyers that your practice is really worth their investment. Compile a comprehensive business presentation package (also referred to as the Business Prospectus) for your practice (Fig. 17–3). The package represents your practice's resume and should include a current valuation report (formal or informal representation of how you decided on the value of the practice), history of the business, description of how the practice operates, description of the facilities, review of the services and products, description of the personnel, identification of the owners, pending legal matters, and 3 to 5 years of financial statements. Prospective buyers will want to see this prospectus, fixed asset inventory, and the financial reports for your practice.

The main components of the prospectus include:

- The history and background of the practice. Include the mission or purpose of the practice, ownership history, marketing niches, strengths of present owners, and a projection of the future of the practice.

- A generic description of the location of the practice (e.g., northeast section of town, on major roadway, within 5 minutes' drive to four hospitals).

- Describe the physical assets, an overview of equipment and supplies. Also include a description of leased or owned facilities.

- Describe the operations of the business of your practice. Include the hours open, sales flow (seasonal?), advertising, public relations, and unusual characteristics of your practice.

- Include a listing of your employees with their titles and salaries. List the benefits your employees are currently receiving. If you know which employees are interested in staying on after the practice sells, you may want to mention who is available for interviews.

- Include a cautionary statement indicating that the patients and employees are not aware that the practice is for sale.

- Define your target market and, if your records allow, give a breakdown of the target market (e.g., average age, distance from practice, income bracket).

- Address the competition briefly and honestly.

- Include your reason for selling. Be careful with your wording in this section. Try to keep it positive.

- The price and terms of the sale should be included.

- Describe the current accounting system you are using and who is doing the day to day bookkeeping as well as the name of your accountant.

- Outline the process for setting up personal interviews.
- Be sure to have your attorney review the prospectus before you print and distribute this document. Your attorney may make changes that may protect you in the long run.

Have your accountant prepare financial reports to show prospective buyers. These numbers verify to buyers that they are buying a profitable practice. A balance sheet gives a snapshot view of the practice's finances on a specific date. Buyers may want to review the past 3 to 5 years of income tax returns. They may also want to see accountant-prepared profit and loss statements.

You should also take the time to make sure the other records of your practice are in order. Some of the records you should evaluate include:

- Articles of incorporation and minutes of directors' and shareholders' meetings
- All governmental agency documents (e.g., OSHA, Medicare, Medicaid)
- Up-to-date tax records. Make sure you are not delinquent with any taxes.
- Leases and contracts
- Payroll records
- Licenses (city, county, biohazard, professional)
- Bank records
- All bookkeeping

Be prepared to share the above information to all serious buyers. Having reviewed the records and having them close at hand will give you a good feeling of confidence when showing your practice. Traditionally, small business owners are known for sloppy record keeping—don't let it be you.

PROFESSIONAL ASSISTANCE

You will be relying on professionals to assist you in preparing and completing the sale of your practice. If you do not already have solid trusting relationships with the needed professionals, do your homework and find some professionals you can trust. Ask colleagues, friends, and family who have sold small businesses in the past for referrals. Even if you do have working relationships with an attorney and accountant, ask them about their history in preparing the needed documents. If they feel uncomfortable (or inexperienced) working on the sale, ask them for a referral. It is much better to know from the start that you have an experienced, well-qualified team of professionals on your side.

Attorney—An attorney should be consulted before you start your preparations for the sale. An attorney can give you guidance and

Figure 17-3	Sample Business Prospectus

Confidential
Business Prospectus
(For the exclusive use of qualified prospective buyers)

A Solo Gynecology Practice

Additional information will be provided *only* after telephone or personal conversations confirm serious interests of both parties. Call (954) 555-5555 between 9 a.m. and 9 p.m.

History and Background

This independent gynecology practice was established in January, 1994. The practice provides gynecological care to women throughout the life span. At a time when much of the medical community felt that the days of independent practice were over, this practice has enjoyed success. The practice has shown geometrical growth every year since opening. This practice is unique in that it was designed as a "cash practice"—meaning, no insurance and no HMOs. Approximately 3% of the patients seen are on Medicaid. Which means, 97% of the patients pay with cash, checks, and credit cards on the day of service. No credit is extended to the patients, so therefore, there are no receivables. There are no insurance companies or HMOs controlling the practice or prescriptions written.

The owner of this practice has gained nationwide recognition for her entrepreneurial expertise. This and other medical expertise has opened many doors for speaking, teaching, research, and other business opportunities.

Due to these opportunities and obligations, the owner chose to see patients only $^3/_4$ of the potential work days in 1998. Even without a full time commitment annual revenues have continued to increase geometrically year after year.

The practice has over 3,000 patient charts with the majority being female, but many males have utilized the laboratory testing services.

Location and Area

The practice is located in the Northeast area of Ft. Lauderdale. Holy Cross Hospital is across the street and three other hospitals are only 10 minutes away. The office condominium is visible from the street and the signage can be read from the street at night. The practice is located on Federal Highway, which is the main street of Ft. Lauderdale. The parking out front is ample and employee parking is in back.

Physical Assets

This is a turn-key business—ready to go. The business office is fully equipped with furniture, computer, printer, Fax, phones, refrigerator and much more. All of the medical furniture and equipment is paid for and is in good repair. The owner's office is very nice with quality office furniture. The entire condo is clean, comfortable, and well maintained. The condominium's current floor plan includes a waiting room, front office, two exam rooms, laboratory, consultation office, and two bathrooms. The condo is approximately 1100 square feet and the current rent being paid is $1400/month.

Figure 17-3 **Sample Business Prospectus** *(Continued)*

Operation

The basic hours of operation are 8:30–5:30, Monday through Friday. In the first year of operation the practice was advertised in several newspapers and mailers. Since then, our patients have found us through the Yellow Pages, and referrals (patients, physicians, and clinics). For the past year, a continuous advertising campaign has been run in a South Florida weekly paper promoting screening for sexually transmitted diseases. This campaign has been very successful in bringing patients into the practice.

The practice is mostly office gynecology, including some special procedures (e.g., colposcopy, cryosurgery, Norplant, sclerotherapy). The revenues of the practice are generated from patient charges, research income, herbal supplement sales, and book sales (written by owner).

Employees

The practice has been run with only one other employee other than the owner for the past 6 years. The employee is one very competent and energetic office manager who has been paid approximately $10/hour; she has insurance through her husband's employer.

Important

The potential sale of the practice has not been announced to patients, suppliers, competitors, or the community. It could be detrimental to the future of the practice for potential sale to be announced prematurely. A buyer under contract to purchase this business will receive full cooperation of the owner in facilitating appropriate exploration.

Competition

There are several other gynecology practices in the area; however, their clientele is more of the insured patient versus the mostly uninsured seen at this practice. Because most of the patients are uninsured and paying cash, the low patient charges have been attracting the patients. Many patients have remarked that they prefer a female provider.

This practice has a lot of room for growth. By adding family practice or obstetrics and/or surgical revenues to the established cash base, one could enjoy a very nice income.

Owners' Reason for Selling

The practice has been put on the market due to the owner's future relocation out of state.

Financial Statements

The bookkeeping for the practice has been performed by the office manager. She has consulted with the CPA as needed. She completes the sales and payroll tax forms as required. For the first 5 years, the practice utilized the simple bookkeeping program *Quicken* and did not have financial statements prepared. The CPA completed the annual tax forms from information submitted. In 1999, the program *QuickBooks* was installed and has been used all year. Financial Reports were not prepared in the prior years.

To arrange to tour the facility and discuss purchasing the practice, please call 954-555-5555 eventually prepare the sale documents. You want an attorney who is well versed in business law and acquisitions.

Accountant—Hopefully you have developed a good working relationship with a certified public accountant (CPA). And hopefully, your CPA has had experience with small business sales in the past. You will be asking your CPA to provide you with very important and specific financial reports. You will need to obtain copies of the past 3 to 5 years of income tax returns for your corporation.

Business Broker—As in real estate transactions, the broker is usually representing the seller—and is paid by the seller. If the deal falls through, the broker does not get paid. Brokers typically receive between 8% and 12% of the agreed sale price. As with real estate sales, brokers are not required, but they may be helpful with this transaction. Brokers may contact your chief competitors, other potential buyers, and advertise your practice for you.

Escrow Company—An escrow company is a business acting as a neutral party that facilitates the collection and preparation of all sale papers. An escrow company can be used instead of a corporate attorney. So, you can work through either your attorney or an escrow company for the closing coordination and documents for the sale of your practice.

VALUING YOUR PRACTICE

This can be a very difficult and possibly the most emotional task you must complete before putting your practice up for sale. Just as beauty is in the eye of the beholder, your practices value is determined by the interest it generates with potential buyers. Unfortunately, what you may think your practice is worth may not be what the buyers are willing to pay. So, arriving at a realistic value of your practice may come with time—seeing and hearing the response of potential buyers.

There are many different formulas available to use to arrive at your asking price for your practice. It seems that every book and everyone you speak with on the subject of selling a small business has a different and unique formula for determining the sale price. In the end, you are basically going to be able to sell your practice for what the market will bear. In other words, what will the buyer spend and how much will you let your practice go for?

The *price* and the *value* of your practice are not the same. Your practice is worth different amounts to the different potential buyers. Many factors come into play during a sale of a business, such as the current market, contract terms, egos, negotiation, financing conditions, and even world events. Your practice can be considered saleable as long as you have a prospective buyer. If you don't have a buyer, then your practice is only worth the liquidation value. No single number will be absolutely correct—so don't let this process bog you down.

It may be beneficial for you to have your practice appraised by a profes-sional. Through the Institute of Business Appraisers (*www.instbusapp.com*) you can locate a directory of business appraisers. Also, the American Institute of Certified Public Accountants (*www.aicpa.org*) has a listing on their Website of CPAs who have a current ABV (Accredited in Business Valuation) certificate. These professionals may be able to assist you in arriving at a value for your practice that is considered reasonable to both you and your prospective buy-ers. It will give your asking price more credibility if a professional calculates the price. Prospective buyers will ask "And how did you arrive at your asking price?" Instead of responding with "It sounded like a good number to me," being able to hand over a professionally prepared appraisal of your practice may help you realize your goal of selling your practice for its full value. An appraisal of your practice will usually cost between $500 and $2,000.

FINDING A BUYER

Now that you have determined a value for your practice and have prepared a presentation package, you are ready to initiate the process of finding an appro-priate buyer for your practice. Like selling a house, it only takes one person to be the right buyer. It could be the first person that inquires about your practice or it may take interacting with several potential buyers until you find the right person. You want to sell your practice as quickly as possible once it is on the market. That is why it is so important to have your practice valued correctly. If for some reason your first price is too high, you may pass up several poten-tial buyers while you learn what the market will bear in regard to a fair price for your practice. You don't want to lose a valid, qualified, prospective buyer because you overpriced your practice. Even if a prospective buyer rejects your first price, keep the dialogue open so you can go back to them if you lower your price later. Also, ask them what they are prepared to pay—that may give you some guidance if you need to adjust your asking price.

There are many different ways to advertise your practice for sale. One thing to keep in mind is that you may want to be careful how you choose to advertise. Getting the word out to potential buyers is one thing, but announc-ing the upcoming sale to the general public may reduce the value of your prac-tice if your patients and employees leave. So, try to market your practice only to professionals who could be potential buyers—not the general public.

Take some time to think of who your "target market" is for the sale of your practice—nurse practitioners, doctors, midwives, doctors of osteopathy, clini-cal nurse specialists, physician assistants, clinic owners, hospitals, practice management companies, and so on. As the saying goes, "If you want to catch fish, go where the fish are." In other words, advertise directly to your target market. Advertising your practice on the Internet through different professional Websites could bring you some potential buyers. Spreading the word through your colleagues can be your best marketing tool. Go to professional meetings and announce that your practice is up for sale. It may not be someone in attendance who is interested, but an attendee may possibly spread the word to someone he or she knows. Encourage your colleagues to spread the word to professionals who might be interested. Local or regional professional newspapers and newsletters can be a great place for advertising. Also, if you have contacts at the local universities and colleges, let them know your practice is up for sale.

When meeting with prospective buyers, try to get them excited about the future of the practice. Just as with networking, try to get to know the potential buyer. If possible, learn a little about the person before the meeting. Try to learn what the buyer would like to do with your practice in the future so you can steer your conversation in that direction. Sketch out an agenda before the meeting so you will have an organized productive meeting. Most importantly, be as open and honest as possible. A lie or bending of the truth can cost you a potential buyer. Think about how you will answer sensitive questions. To help prepare yourself for the meeting, think about what questions you would ask if you were the buyer and then rehearse your answers.

When creating advertising for your practice, do not use the name of your practice in the advertising piece (Fig. 17–4). Use enough words to get a buyer to call about the ad, but no more than that. Include what type of practice you have to help weed out inappropriate callers.

SHOWING YOUR PRACTICE

Just as if you were preparing your home for sale, you need to prepare your practice to be seen in at its best. Take a pad and pencil and do a walk-through from front to back. Look at your facility with a critical eye. Pretend you are coming in for the first time. First impressions are very important for potential buyers. Write down every little thing that needs repair, paint, patching, replacing, and cleaning. The first few things that a prospective buyer looks at is the general appearance and housekeeping of the practice. If your practice envi-

Figure 17–4   Sample Advertisement

SOLO GYNECOLOGY PRACTICE FOR SALE

This successful cash practice was established in 1994. Owner relocating out of state. Near several quality hospitals. Desirable location in **North East Ft. Lauderdale**. This practice is located in a fully equipped beautiful office that has been well maintained. Property can be included or excluded in the sale. For more information, **please call 954-555-5555**.

ronment is in need of repair and cleaning, it could be a major turn-off to the prospective buyer. Depending on the air quality of your office, you may want to invest in some type of air freshener, so your office not only looks clean and fresh but also smells clean and fresh. Take a good look at the exterior of the building. Pick up any garbage in the parking area and surrounding the building. Check for needed repairs and updates.

Once you have done these repairs and cleaning, you are ready to show your practice with pride. When appointments are scheduled with prospective buyers, take the time to tidy up so they can see your facility at its best.

You should have all of the written materials regarding the sale of your practice handy. If the potential buyer has received the prospectus before your appointment, he or she may have questions, and it will be easier to address the questions with your paperwork in front of you.

NEGOTIATIONS

As with most things, preparation is key. Learn as much as possible about prospective buyers. Look at the transaction from his or her perspective. Try to anticipate their objectives and negotiating style, as well as leverage points that can be used in your favor.

Take the time and really think about what you need and want from the sale of your practice. The "needs," of course, are necessities, and the "wants" are not necessary but would be nice. Keeping that list in sight during the negotiations may help you stay on track. You may be able to identify some of the things that you listed as "wants" to be flexible and might help make the deal if you make concessions. Then again, don't be so eager to make the deal that you give away all of your wants. Try to get something in return when you make a concession, for example, "If I sign the non-compete agreement for 2 years, will you agree to sign a lease for the office I own for three years?"

Negotiating with a potential buyer can be stressful. To help reduce the stress, keep the following tips in mind:

- Prepare before your negotiations—learn as much as possible about the buyer.
- Always negotiate in person—not through e-mails, fax, or telephone calls.
- Keep your emotions in check—this is a business deal.
- Try to be flexible—be ready to make concessions.
- Know what you are willing to give up in the negotiations—have it listed out.
- Keep your eye on your goals—write them down and have them in front of you.
- Use your listening skills—let the buyer talk.

- Be very careful what you say—and also what you ask.

- Always be open and honest—if you lie, they will find out.

- Don't be afraid to walk away from the deal—if the deal doesn't fit your goals, don't agree to it.

- Never walk away from a deal unless you mean it—only after you have exhausted every option should you walk away from a deal.

- Many times, what is important to us in the deal is not quite as important to the buyer. We are concerned with continuity of care, keeping our good name, keeping the practice running under our own model—more of the emotional aspects of the transaction. Whereas, the buyer may look at the deal as more of a dollars and cents type of transaction. He or she is thinking "can I make this practice not only work, but will I make enough money while growing the practice into the practice of *my* dreams?"

FINANCING

Even though the acquisition of financing is the responsibility of the buyer, if you can help the buyer, it may speed up the sale process. You can help the buyer by providing the necessary documents needed if they are applying for traditional financing. The lending institution may look at the past history of the practice, such as: the credit history, existing assets, business goodwill, and more.

There are several financing options for your potential buyer, such as loans from:

- Family
- Friends
- Investors
- Commercial banks
- Credit cards
- Credit lines
- Personal banks
- Small Business Association
- Seller

Most small business owners who are selling their businesses realize that they may need to participate in the buyer's financing of the business. The potential buyer may ask you if you will finance the sale. You need to be ready with an answer. If your answer is "No, I must have all cash," then you will certainly reduce your number of potential buyers. You may want to offer the option that you will finance a percentage of the sale price at a reasonable interest rate. If you insist on an all-cash deal, you may reduce your number of potential prospects by half.

Your attorney or an escrow company needs to be involved in this portion of the sale. The existing assets of the practice may be all the collateral required for owner financing. Traditional lenders usually want to attach personal assets as collateral for the loan. Another option may be to accept cash for the goodwill, business name, and charts—then lease the equipment to the buyer for a fixed amount of time on a lease-purchase contract. Whatever financing arrangement you have made, be sure your attorney or escrow company has drafted the appropriate papers.

FINANCING TERMINOLOGY

Accounts payable—The amount owed to creditors for services and goods.

Accounts receivable—The amount due by patients or customers for services or products.

Accrual—This method of accounting recognizes income and expenses on the basis of when it was earned rather than when the payment was received.

Amortization—The process of gradually paying off amount due over a scheduled time period.

Balance sheet—A brief financial statement that shows what the business owns and owes and what the equity value is on a certain date.

Balloon—Financing conditions in which payouts are based on a long-term basis, but the remaining principal falls due in a shorter time period.

Book value—The net worth of the business. Assets less liabilities, as seen on the business's balance sheet.

Buyer paper—A promissory note from the buyer identifying specific amounts to be paid by the buyer to the seller on specific dates.

Capital (or equity)—The money invested in a business by the owner.

Capital expenditures—Purchases of long-term assets (e.g., furniture, equipment).

Capital gains—Profits from the sale of capital assets.

Cash flow—The cash coming in the business minus the outgoing cash during a defined amount of time.

Closing—The completion of the transaction. The signing of all agreements and change of ownership.

Covenants—Included in letter of intent or the purchase contract. This is an agreement to perform or abstain from certain activities. These can be directed to either the buyer or the seller.

Depreciation—The amortization of the cost of a fixed asset over its projected years of use.

Due diligence—An exploration done by the buyer to confirm what is being offered is really what is being sold. Data must be true, accurate, and complete.

Fixed (or hard) assets—Equipment, furniture, fixtures—anything tangible—owned by a business.

Fixed costs—Expenses of the business that don't vary; also referred to as "overhead."

Goodwill—An intangible asset. It is the perceived value of the company's name, reputation, and anticipated future earnings. Goodwill can have an assigned value.

Intangible assets—These assets are not related to a physical thing. See Goodwill.

Inventory—Supplies and goods.

Letter of intent—A non-binding summary of what has been agreed upon regarding the sale of the business.

Net income—The profit that is left after all expenses are deducted from the gross income.

Net worth—The excess of assets after deducting the liabilities.

Non-compete covenant—language contained in a legal document that states that for a specific number of years, the seller will not enter into business that will hinder or detract from the business sold.

Operating expenses—The cost of running your practice. Day to day expenses.

Present value—The current value of payments due.

Prime rate—This is the interest rate that banks give their most favored customers.

Principal—Unpaid balance remaining on a loan.

Pro forma—Projected income statement showing anticipated revenues, costs, and expenses over a specific period of time.

Prospectus—A concise description of the business that offers enough information for preliminary review.

Seller financing—The seller holds a portion or all of the price financed.

Service business—The business is more one of providing labor than one that sells or produces products.

Term note—Interest-bearing debt that is due on a certain date.

Valuation—The art and science of estimating the most likely price that will be accepted by buyers and sellers alike.

THE CLOSING

The closing is the actual consummation of the transaction through the execution of all documents and the transfer of title in exchange for a transfer of funds. Ideally, the closing should be quick, well organized, and a pleasant experience in which you sign the final documents, hand over the keys, and wish each other well! However, if things have not been thoroughly discussed and misunderstandings are possible, it can become a tense, lengthy, and unpleasant experience.

The responsibility of the seller in regard to the closing is to have all the papers signed, documents gathered, loans approved, and leases assigned. Get all this in order as soon as possible. Your attorney or escrow company will help you with the closing. Be sure to give all requested documents quickly. Follow up regularly with the buyers and your attorney. If a problem or question arises, deal with it immediately. If for some reason the deal falls through, you need to know as soon as possible so you can resume marketing your practice for sale.

TRANSITION

The transition of ownership for a health-care practice can be a sensitive issue. It is really up to the buyer's wants and needs and what you feel comfortable with providing. Some buyers may want you to stay on as an employee for a certain rate of pay for a certain amount of time, whereas some buyers may want you to quietly disappear.

Before you sign any agreements, be sure to check with your lawyers regarding the state laws for selling a practice. There may be required notices you need to publish in the newspapers. You may have to send letters to different organizations (Board of Nursing, Board of Medicine, Medicare, Medicaid, insurance companies). You may be required to notify your patients of the change in ownership. These requirements vary from state to state.

You may want to work with the buyer to compose a letter to your patients that introduces the new provider to the practice. It may be unpleasant for a patient to call and think he or she is scheduling an appointment with you and then arrive to find a new provider.

SUGGESTIONS AND TIPS FROM WOMEN'S HEALTH WATCH, INC.

- Once the preparations for the sale were complete, the practice was listed for sale in every possible place on the Internet, newsletters, newspapers, and journals. After many interviews and meetings, the practice was sold to someone who heard about the practice from a friend! The friend was a colleague who also referred patients to Women's Health Watch.

■ The valuation of the practice was not professionally done and as a result was initially way out of line. Through trial and error, a workable price was finally agreed upon. How many potential buyers did the incorrect pricing put off? Maybe it would have sold quicker with appropriate pricing.

■ Owner financing was not seriously considered until several potential buyers said that owner financing for a portion of the sale price was necessary. Weighing out the pros and cons of owner financing and having a sharp attorney finally gave me the confidence to carry the financing for 50% of the sale price.

PERSONAL ANECDOTES

1. I was truly not prepared for the emotional component of the sale of my practice. I only anticipated the happy feelings of successfully selling my practice. I felt a true loss (I still do at times) for "my baby." I guess this is normal because I created it and nurtured the practice into a viable and valuable business.

2. I was unsure of my abilities to negotiate the sale at first. So I had my CPA come to the first couple of meetings to help guide the negotiations. I learned from her and became more confident that I could negotiate the sale.

3. I can't stress enough how important it is to surround yourself with competent, qualified professionals. I will always be thankful for the help I had during the sale process from my accountant and my attorney. I am lucky enough to call them both friends and trust them with my life (and livelihood!).

Resources

American Institute of Certified Public Accountants: *www.aicpa.org.*
CCH Business Owner's Tool Kit: Small business financing: How and where to get it. Chicago, CCH Incorporated, 1998.
Conroy, H: Let's make a deal: What you should know about negotiating contracts. Enterprising Women 5:38–39, 2001.
Curren, AM: (2001). Selling your business. Enterprising Women 5:50–52, 2001.
Gabriel, C: How to sell your business—and get what you want! A pragmatic guide with revealing tips from 57 sellers. Westport, CT, Gwent Press, 1998.
Hekman, KM: Buying, selling and merging a medical practice: Proven valuation and negotiation strategies. Toronto: Irwin Professional Publishing, 1997.
Horn, TW: Unlocking the value of your business: How to increase it, measure it and negotiate an actual sale price in easy step-by-step terms. New York, Charter Oaks Press, 1999.
Institute of Business Appraisers: *www.instbusapp.org.*

Small Business Administration: *www.sba.gov*.

Sperry, PS, and Mitchell, BH: The complete guide to selling your business. Dover, NH, Upstart Publishing Company, 1992.

Tuller, LW: Getting out: A step-by-step guide to selling a business or professional practice. New York, Liberty Hall Press, 1990.

Tuller, LW: The small business valuation book. Holbrook, MA, Adams Media Corporation, 1998.

Umbenhauer, RE: Sell your business successfully: Tips, strategies, and tools. New York, John Wiley and Sons, 1999.

Yegge, WM: A basic guide for buying and selling a company. New York, John Wiley and Sons, 1996.

Yegge, WM: A basic guide for valuing a company. New York, John Wiley and Sons, 1996.

N O T E S

Chapter 18

Conclusions and Recommendations: Should I Really Do It?

" Make the most of yourself, for that is all there is of you "

Ralph Waldo Emerson

Making the commitment to start your own practice may be one of the biggest decisions you ever make. This book should help you in making this decision. Is your desire for an independent practice stronger than your fear of failure?

From personal experience, starting my own practice was one of the best decisions I ever made. My practice gave me independence, autonomy, control, satisfaction, financial reward, fun, and a new identity in the community as a health care provider and business owner. I provided care to my patients in a wonderful environment that I created and controlled.

During the decision-making process of whether to open my practice, I did the math. I tried to estimate how much money I could potentially lose in a year. Once I came up with that number, I had to laugh—my brothers owed me more than that! That exercise helped me put my financial risks in perspective. If the business failed, I would just have another brother!

If I had the opportunity to do it over again, I would. Is it right for you? Everyone's situation is different. Weighing your family and financial commitments is probably the most important consideration.

If you do decide to start your own practice, I wish you the best of luck.

Web Directory

ADP (automatic data processing)—*www.adp.com* or 1-800-225-5237

All-in-One Directory, Gebbie Press, Inc.—*www.gebbieinc.com*

American Academy of Family Physicians, patient education handouts—
www.familydoctor.org

American Academy of Nurse Practitioners—*www.aanp.org*

American Association of Legal Nurse Consultants—*www.aalnc.org*

American Institute of Certified Public Accountants—*www.aicpa.org*

American Medical Association—*www.ama-assn.org*

American Nurses Publishing—*www.nursesbooks.org*

Americans with Disabilities Act. Information—*www.usdoj.gov/crt/ada/adahom1.htm*

Background check companies—www.repchceck.com, www.knowx.com, www.informus.com, and *www.confi-chek.com*

Bacon's Media Catalog—*www.baconsinfo.com*

Best's Guide to Insurance Companies, A. M. Best Company—*www.ambest.com*

Calendars, traditional and nontraditional recognition days—*www.chases.com*

Ccnow, internet credit card processing—*www.ccnow.com*

Certified Financial Planners Directory—*www.fpanet.org/plannersearch/index.cfm*

Chic Ideas, Inc., Novelties—*www.chicideas.com* or 954-587-5316

Child labor laws—*www.dol.gov*

Clinical Research Investigator Registry—*www.criregistry.com*

Computer purchasing info, International Computer Negotiations—*www.dobetterdeals.com*

Contemporary Health Communications—*http://patient-info.com* or 1-800-234-1742

Dale Carnegie Courses—*www.westcgg.com*

Darby Drug Company—*www.darbydrug.com*

Department of Health and Human Services Hot Tips—*Htipds@os.dhhs.gov*

Drug Enforcement Administration—*www.DEAdiversions.usdoj.gov*

Employer Identification Number information—*http://www.irs.gov/forms_pubs/pubs/p58303.htm*

FA Davis Company—*www.fadavis.com* or 1-800-323-3555

Federal Bureau of Investigation—*www.fbi.gov*

Florida Infusion, prescription medication sales—*www.floridainfusion.com* or 727-942-1829

Florida Patient's Bill of Rights—*http://www.doh.state.fl.us/mqa/profiling/billofrights.htm*

Frisk-E-Business, free marketing e-zine—*Heidi@FriskEBusiness.com*

HIPA Advisory—*www.hipaadvisory.com*

ImageCafe, Inc., Web page design—*www.imagecafe.com*

Institute of Business Appraisers—*www.instbusapp.org*

Insurance Broker, B&B Coverage LTD—*www.bbcoverage.com* or 516-872-2300

IRS electronic filing information—*http://www.irs.gov/elec_svc/efile-bus.html* or 512-460-8900

Kaplan College—*www.kaplancollege.edu/LN* or 1-800-669-2555

LiveCapital corporate—*www.livecapital.com/getfinancing.html*

Malpractice insurance information, NP Central Website—*www.nurse.net*

Media Guide to Health Care Experts, Sigma Theta Tau International—*www.nursingsociety.org*

Media Networks, Inc., major advertising opportunities—*www.medianetworks.com*

Medical Software Reviews Newsletter—www.healthcarecomputing.com

Medical-Legal Consulting Institute—*www.legalnurse.com* or 1-800-880-0944

Medicare Anti-Kickback Statute—*www.complianceland.com/aks/fedreg-7-29-91.html*

Medicomp—*www.erols.com*

Medicserve—*www.medicserve.com*

Medisoft—*www.medisoft.com*

Medline*plus—http://www.medlineplus.gov*

National Association of Women Business Owners (NAWBO)—*www.nawbo.org*

National Committee for Quality Assurance (NCQA)—*www.ncqa.org*

National Institutes of Health—*www.clinicalstudies.info.nih.gov*

National Practitioner Data Bank—*www.npdb.com* or 1-800-767-6732

National Procedures Institute—*www.NPInstitute* or 1-800-462-2492

Nationtax Online (Form 941 electronic filing)—*http://www.nationtax.com* or 1-877-786-3453

Nationwide Hospital Insurance Billing Directory, Francis B. Kelly—*http://www.fbka.com*

NCLEX—*www.ncsbn.org* or 312-787-6555 extension 496

Newspaper links—*www.webwombat.com.au/intercom/newsprs/index.htm*

NP Central: brochures, directory sample letter and registry—*www.nurse.net*

NP Central—*http://www.nurse.net/npcentral*

NP Clinics, registry—*www.npclinics.com*

OSHA Guidelines for workplace violence—*www.osha.gov* or 202-693-1888

Patient Care for the Nurse Practitioner—*www.patientcarenp.com*

Paychex—*www.paychex.com* or 1-800-322-7292

PayPal—*www.paypal.com*

Pharmaceutical Research and Manufacturers of America—*www.phrma.org/patients*

Physician's Payment Update (February 2001)—*http://www.ahcpub.com/online.html*

Physicians Total Care, automated medication dispensing system—*www.physianstotalcare.com*

PlanMagic Corporation—*www.planmagic.com*

PlanWrite for marketing computer software—*www.brs-inc.com*

Publicity Blitz Media Directory—*www.rtir.com*

Pyxis, automated medication dispensing system—*www.pyxis.com*

QuickBooks or QuickBooks Pro by Intuit—*www.quicken.com* or 1-888-2-Intuit

Sell Shareware—*www.SellShareware.com/ProgramInfo.asp?AfID=7838&PrID=34362*

Small Business Administration—*www.sba.gov*

Speak Easy Seminars—*www.speakeasy.net*

Speech Tips—*www.speechtips.com*

Teragenix—*www.teragenix.com*

The Capitol Connection—www.capitolconnection.com

The Small Business Resource Guide—http://www.irs.gov/bus_info/sm_bus/smbus-cd.html

Toastmasters International—www.toastmasters.org

United States Department of Health and Human Services—*www.hhs.gov/ocr/hipaa.html*

United States Small Business Administration—*www.sba.gov*

VeriSign, domain name registration—*www.netsol.com*

Vista Writer's Guide, VistaMedEd—*www.vistameded.com* or 209-476-8673

Women's Health Watch—*www.independentnp.com*

N O T E S

Index

Note: Page numbers followed by "f" refer to illustrations; numbers followed by "t" refer to tables; and numbers followed by "b" refer to boxed material.

Business (*continued*)
  sole proprietor's, 48
  stress associated with, 13
 marketing of. *See* Marketing.
 naming of, 59–60
 niche occupied by, 10–11
  marketing in relation to, 169. *See also* Marketing.
 patients served by, 36, 49. *See also* Patient(s).
 planning of, 9, 11, 46, 47
  written, Women's Health Watch Inc. support for, 51
 sale of. *See* Sale of practice.
 setting goals for, 4, 5f
 site for, 36, 64. *See also* Office.
 start of. *See* Start of practice.
 success of, reasons for, 7
 technologies used in, 268–278
 type of services provided by, deciding on, 36
Business broker, as aid to sale of practice, 294
Business cards, in marketing, 171–172
Business goals, setting of, by nurse practitioner, 4, 5f
Business loans, 70–71
 sources for, websites of, 72b, 73
Business logo, design of, 60
Business owners' insurance, 40, 125
Business plan, 9, 11, 46, 47
 written, Women's Health Watch Inc. support for, 51
Business prospectus, defined, 300
 in sale of practice, 290f–291f, 292–293
Business umbrella insurance policy, 125
Buyer, of practice, 295
  financing for, 298
  negotiations with, 297–298
Buyer paper, defined, 299

C

Calendar-based planning, of business marketing, 165, 166b
Capital (equity), defined, 299
Capital expenditures, defined, 299
Capital gains, defined, 299
Capitation, 105b
"Carve-out," 105b
Case management, 105b
Cash flow, defined, 299
Certification, of laboratory, 67–68
 of nurse practitioner, 27, 28t
Certified public accountant (CPA), recruitment of, 220, 222
 support from, 59
 in sale of practice, 294
CEUs (Continuing Education Units), 26
Chart(s). *See* Medical record(s).
Claim form, for health insurance, 95f
Claims-made policies, 120
Cleaning, of office, responsibility for, 40
CLIA (Clinical Laboratory Improvement Act), 67
Clinical Laboratory Improvement Act (CLIA), 67
Clinical research, by independent nurse practitioner, 261–262
Closed panel model, of managed health plan, 105b
Closing, defined, 299
 in sale of practice, 301

Coding, 109–110
Collaborating physician, 78–81
 liability of, 85
 payment of, 41, 80–81
 role of, notification of Board of Medicine regarding, 61, 61b
 Women's Health Watch Inc. experiences with, 86–87
Collateral, 71
Collateral (marketing collateral), 171–177
Comment cards, patient survey by, 210–211, 212f
Communication, with patients, 239–247
 via e-mail, 275–276
 via telephone, 241–242
  Women's Health Watch Inc. approach to, 246
Communication skills, 18–19
 exploitation of, by independent nurse practitioner, 251–253
Community method, of establishing capitation rates, 105b
Compensation, collaborating physician's, 41, 80–81
Competitive medical plan, 105b
Complementary medicine, 263
Computers, 268–272
 purchase of, checklist for, 270f
 Women's Health Watch Inc. tips regarding, 277
Confidentiality, 244–245, 276–277
 inclusion of notices of, with fax transmissions, 176b
Consent, patient, forms for, 147, 148–149, 155f, 161f
Consultant, legal nurse, 255
 marketing, 59
Consultations, 86
Contests, in marketing, 213
Continuing education, 26, 43, 257–258
Contract, employer-employee, 234–235
 insurance policy. *See* Insurance.
Contractor, independent, criteria for, 231f
 vs. employee, 229
Corporation, nursing practice as, 48
Cost estimation (budgeting), for marketing, 41, 182f
 for start of practice, 37–44, 38f
Covenant(s), defined, 299–300
Cover sheets, for faxes, in marketing, 176
CPA (certified public accountant), recruitment of, 220, 222
 support from, 59
 in sale of practice, 294
CPT (Current Procedural Terminology) code, 105b, 110
Current Procedural Terminology (CPT) code, 105b, 110
Curriculum vitae (CV), development of, 20, 22, 23f–25f
 updating of, Women's Health Watch Inc. endorsement of, 29, 32

D

DEA (Drug Enforcement Administration), 137–138
Deductions, IRS, 225–226
Denial, of hospital privileges, 133
 persistence of record of, 131

N

Naming, of business practice, 59–60
National Association of Women Business
  Owners (NAWBO), 74
National certification, of nurse practitioners, 27
National Committee on Quality Assurance
  (NCQA), 107b
National health observance events, 190b–199b
National Practitioner Data Bank (NPDB), 123
NAWBO (National Association of Women
  Business Owners), 74
NCQA (National Committee on Quality
  Assurance), 107b
Negligence, 116
Net income, defined, 300
Net worth, defined, 300
Network model HMO, 107b
Networking, in marketing, 177–181
  websites of national organizations for, 177b
Newsletters, in marketing, 204–205
Newspapers, in marketing, 185
Niche (business niche), for solo practice, 10–11
  marketing in relation to, 169. *See also*
    Marketing.
Non-complete covenant, defined, 300
Nontraditional marketing, 187, 189–190
Nonverbal communication, 19
Novelties, advertising, as marketing tools, 211
NPDB (National Practitioner Data Bank), 123
Nurse consultant, legal, 255
Nurse practitioner(s). *See also* Independent
    nurse practitioner.
  certification of, 27, 28t
  goal-setting by, 4, 5f
  independent. *See* Independent nurse
    practitioner.
  journals for, 29, 31t–32t
  organizations for, 29, 30t
    dues charged by, 43
  scope of services provided by, 22, 26, 81
  self-assessment by, 3–4
    business goals in, 4, 5f
    personal goals in, 4, 5f
    personal strengths and weaknesses in, 7, 8f
  self-employed. *See* Independent nurse
    practitioner.
Nursing education, continuing, 26, 43, 257–258

O

Occupational risk, of violence, 235
  reduction of, 235–236
Occupational Safety and Health Act (OSHA),
  68
Occurrence-based liability insurance, 120
Office, 36–41, 65–66. *See also* Business.
  costs relating to, estimation of, 39, 40
  safety of, 73–74
  site of, 36
Office procedure–related income, opportunities
  for increases in, 259f–260f
Office space, leasing of, as source of extra
  income, 257
  leasing vs. purchasing of, 65
Online pharmacies, 139
Open enrollment period, 107b
Open panel model, of managed health plan,
  107b

Open-house invitation, in marketing, 207, 207f
Operating expenses, defined, 300
Organizations/associations, for nurse
  practitioners, 29, 30t
  dues charged by, 43
OSHA (Occupational Safety and Health Act), 68
Ownership, transition of, in sale of practice, 301

P

Partial risk, 107b
Partnership, in business, 48
Part-time work, as source of extra income, 251
Patient(s), 36, 49
  appointment cards for, 173, 173f
  appointment reminders for, 173
  appointment scheduling for, 242
  birthday cards for, 208
  communication with, 239–247
    via e-mail, 275–276
    via telephone, 241–242
      Women's Health Watch Inc. approach to,
      246
  consent forms for, 147, 148–149, 155f, 161f
  data sheet ("welcome form") for, in medical
    records, 147, 153f
  drug advertisements directed at, 244
  education of, 243
  e-mail communication with, 275–276
  family history of, recording of, 146–147, 152f
  health insurance disclosure restrictions relating
    to, 245, 277
  insurance providers covering, 94
    payment from, 94, 96
  interview with, documentation of, 148, 158f
  medical record of. *See* Medical record(s).
  payments from or made by insurers of, 89–96
  personal history of, recording of, 146–147,
    152f
  physical examination of, recording results of,
    147, 154f
  prescription record of, charting of, 147–148,
    156f
  privacy rights of, 244–245, 276–277
    inclusion of notices of, with fax
      transmissions, 176b
  problem, 122
  release of information regarding, 148, 149–150,
    159f
  survey of, via comment cards, 210–211, 212f
  telephone communication with, 241–242
    Women's Health Watch Inc. approach to, 246
  termination of relationship with, 245–246
  tests of, follow-up systems for, 149
  written agreement of, to drug prescription
    policy, 142f
Patient consent, forms for, 147, 148–149, 155f,
  161f
Patient data sheet ("welcome form"), 147, 153f
Patient history, recording of, 146–147, 152f
Patient interview sheet, 148, 158f
Patient records. *See* Medical record(s).
Payment, collaborating physician's, 41, 80–81
Payroll, 42
Payroll taxes, 42, 224–225
Per diem work, as source of extra income, 251
Personal goals, setting of, by nurse practitioner,
  4, 5f